W9-BYY-809

The Psychological
Consultant

The Psychological Consultant

Edited by

Jerome J. Platt, Ph.D.

Professor of Mental Health Sciences
Hahnemann Medical College and Hospital
Philadelphia, Pennsylvania

Robert J. Wicks, Psy.D.

Assistant Professor
The Graduate School of Social Work and Social Research
Bryn Mawr College
Bryn Mawr, Pennsylvania

Grune & Stratton
A Subsidiary of Harcourt Brace Jovanovich, Publishers
New York   London   Toronto   Sydney   San Francisco

Library of Congress Cataloging in Publication Data
Main entry under title:

The Psychological consultant.

    Includes bibliographies and index.
    1. Psychological consultation. I. Platt,
Jerome J. II. Wicks, Robert J. [DNLM: 1. Counsel-
ing. 2. Consultants. 3. Psychology. WM55 P974]
BF637.C56P75   658.4'6   79-9186
ISBN 0-8089-1187-2

Grune & Stratton, Inc.
111 Fifth Avenue
New York, New York 10003

Distributed in the United Kingdom by
Academic Press, Inc. (London) Ltd.
24/28 Oval Road, London NW 1

Library of Congress Catalog Number 79-9186
International Standard Book Number 0-8089-1187-2

Printed in the United States of America

Contents

Preface

Although psychologists have functioned as consultants in a variety of settings, consulting was once considered to be outside the mainstream of professional psychological activity. Recent years, however, have been marked by a growing demand for the psychological consultant's services in education, business, government, industry, criminal justice, and public health. Psychologists are becoming more involved in full-time and part-time consultant work as the job market in traditional academic positions continues to deteriorate. Graduate students and experienced professionals alike are demonstrating greater interest in consulting as employment opportunities expand. Consultants are filling essential roles as advisors and facilitators of research and clinical intervention in an increasingly broad range of settings.

In the role of consultant, the psychologist often deals with subjects not traditionally taught in graduate school and in which the tools and skills of the psychologist may not be perfectly understood. Novice consultants often may encounter resistance, especially among their clients' employees. To date, there is unfortunately little literature specifically directed to answering questions about the consulting process—questions which range from the broadly theoretical to the more practical ("How do I handle *this* situation?"). These are precisely the questions the present volume is designed to address. Issues of expertise acquisition and types of activities, as well as the current status and expected future trends of consultation in the areas of education, industry, government, police work, courts, and correctional agencies are discussed. Finally, two crucial areas—dealing with paraprofessionals and designing adequate evaluation components—are covered in some detail. This volume thus provides a thorough introduction to the theory and practice of psychological consultation. It meets the expanding needs and interests both of students and of licensed psychologists who are seeking more information on opportunities and methodologies available to the psychological consultant.

The opportunities for consultation are not limited to those described in this book; we look forward to substantial changes in future research and theory development. In the meantime, we feel our selection of representative areas, in which the demand for psychological consultants is either well established or rapidly growing, offers concrete information to the psychologist wishing to explore new career opportunities.

Jerome J. Platt, Ph.D.
Robert J. Wicks, Psy.D.

Contributors

D. A. Andrews, Ph.D.
Associate Professor
Carlton University
Ottawa, Canada

Alphonse Buccino, Ph.D.
Director
Office of Program Integration
National Science Foundation
Washington, D.C.

Thomas D. Cook, Ph.D.
Professor
Northwestern University
Evanston, Illinois

Darwin Dorr, Ph.D.
Chief Psychologist and Associate Professor
Highland Hospital
Division of Duke University Medical Center
Asheville, North Carolina

C. Abraham Fenster, Ph.D.
Professor
Department of Psychology
John Jay College of Criminal Justice
The City University of New York
New York, New York

Eugenie Walsh Flaherty, Ph.D.
Director of Research and Evaluation
Philadelphia Health Management Corporation
Philadelphia, Pennsylvania

Paul Gendreau, Ph.D.
Regional Co-ordinating Psychologist
Ontario Ministry of Correctional Services
Rideau Correctional Centre
Burritt's Rapids, Ontario

Florence W. Kaslow, Ph.D.
Professor
Hahnemann Medical College and Hospital
Philadelphia, Pennsylvania

Theodore Kunin, Ph.D.
Vice President
Psychological Consultants to Industry, Inc.
Pittsburgh, Pennsylvania

Christina Labate
Fellow in Psychiatry
University of Chicago
Department of Human Development
Chicago, Illinois

Jonathan A. Morell, Ph.D.
Assistant Professor
Hahnemann Medical College and Hospital
Philadelphia, Pennsylvania

Marshall Sashkin, Ph.D.
Senior Editorial Associate
University Associates, Publishers, and Consultants
San Diego, California

Harvey Schlossberg, Ph.D.
Adjunct Associate Professor
John Jay College of Criminal Justice
The City University of New York
New York, New York

The Psychological
Consultant

Jerome J. Platt,
Robert J. Wicks,
Christina Labate

1
The Psychological Consultant

It has been suggested that the distressing lack of knowledge about the process of consultation is in part a consequence of the characteristics of consultants themselves:

> The consultants are in the "practicing professions"—those individuals who are constantly "doing." They are usually not interested in research in general, or research around the nature of their consultation activities in particular. . . . They are often unable to . . . conduct this kind of evaluation or research program themselves . . . , [and] the nature of most . . . consulting contracts [does] not lend [itself] to this kind of research activity (Burke, 1971, p. 483).

At the most basic level, the very abundance of definitions of "consultation" reflects the variety in types of consultant – client relationships—each of which is directed to achieving apparently equally various immediate objectives. These definitions have also been termed "models" of consultation in an effort to systematize a largely chaotic accumulation of subjective and objective impressions. A brief review of some of the major thinking on these issues will provide an introduction to the process of consultation.

Models of Consultation

In broadest terms, consultation has been said to have as its goal the improvement of clients' use of their capabilities and resources to achieve their objectives (Smith & Sorenson, 1974). Consultants themselves will vary tremendously with respect to experience, technical ability, reputation, and sophistication, but in each case they will be operating to some extent with the above-mentioned goal in mind. A review of the literature on the process of consultation yields a variety of models in which the phrases and categories proposed differ according to the writer's professional perspective; yet it can be argued that, despite apparent diversity and irreconcilability among these various models, at the most fundamental level each represents a serious attempt to grapple with this common, essential, underlying goal. In one respect, then, these models are but variations on a theme. Consequently, their diversity becomes more manageable and comprehensible to the novice.

One useful method of viewing consultant−client relationships is organized around the three general types of services a consultant may be asked to provide: (1) handling a problem the client knows little about (e.g., giving expert advice); (2) providing an independent opinion, particularly in the case where the client cannot be reasonably expected to have an unbiased opinion; and (3) providing additional expertise in an area familiar to the client but one that the client lacks adequate resources to handle (Jacoby, 1974). To some extent the psychological consultant will experience at various times a demand for each of the above services; however, it should not be inferred that the three services are mutually exclusive. In fact, as will be seen later, there is often considerable overlap in these three types of services.

A slightly different classification scheme is offered by Burke (1971) from the perspective of the consultant−organization client relationship. In this context, consulting may be categorized first as a simple "purchase−sale transaction." What is purchased is expert information or services tailored to meet some specific need of the client. This type of structured relationship is most useful when the client is more in need of information than of help, since the "purchaser" in this case determines what his actual needs are. In a second case, consulting may be viewed more as a reciprocal and continuous flow of information between client and consultant. Burke (1971) points out that often a relationship of this type may prove to be inadequate if there is no provision for converting such information into constructive activity. A third and perhaps more useful type of relationship involves "process consultation," in which joint diagnosis of the problem is undertaken. The consultant's role is to teach the client problem-solving skills and to generate and explore alternative solutions in order to enable the client to reach an educated decision.

The consultant has been viewed by many as primarily a change agent who may only indirectly deal with a specific problem situation while directly dealing with those individuals involved in it (Bindman, 1966). In the case where the consultant is also a psychologist, the nature of the change effected may specifically involve human behavior, whether at the level of attitudes and perceptions, interpersonal relations, or services provided. Usually, the consultant−client relationship is concerned exclusively with the work-related problem of the client, and the process is exceedingly goal-directed. Many reviewers have commented on the fact that the consultant is usually an "outsider" who is temporarily involved with the client's work system for the purpose of helping the client with specific problems falling within the consultant's specialized area of expertise (Bindman, 1966; Burke, 1971; Pearl, 1974; Smith & Sorenson, 1974). The consultant is often expected to be of assistance both in identifying general problems and in outlining alternative solutions. Along this spectrum of objectives consultants can be asked to (1) define problems, (2) determine if consultation can be of help in dealing with those problems, (3) analyze alternative solutions, (4) recommend the best solution for each particular client, and (5) assist in implementing the action agreed upon (Smith & Sorenson, 1974).

Content of Consultation

The specific content of consultation will, of course, vary with the client's needs and stated preferences; the interaction can, at times, border on education, supervision, psychotherapy, administration, and collaboration, although these are not strictly considered to be functions of consultation per se (Bindman, 1966). While a secondary goal of consultation is often education, the long-term commitment in which content is formally planned is lacking (Bindman, 1966). Particularly in the case of a clinical psychologist consulting to a mental health system, the nature of the relationship between consultant and client can unwittingly approach that of psychotherapy. However, Bindman (1966) is cautious to point out that the consultant is not there to *treat* the consultee and hence should only deal indirectly with personal problems. Rather, in each transaction, ideally "the consultant utilizes the consultation process to improve the consultee's own professional skills in handling mental health predicaments" (Bindman, 1966, p. 82).

Phases of Consultation

Irrespective of specific content, there are a number of characteristic phases to the consultation process. Generally, the period immediately prior to the initiation of consultant contact is one in which the potential client is assessing the problem and evaluating the resources available for meeting it. Once the consultant is contacted, a "preparatory" or "entry" phase is reached in which client and consultant discuss the need for consultation, explore the bases on which an agreement can be reached, and outline a contract detailing the services and functions expected of both parties. In the next phase further development of the consultant−client relationship occurs. At this point the consultant is beginning to reach some understanding of the client's problems and is actively interacting with the client's employees. It is often useful to engage in group discussion at this point. Often during this phase resistance and misunderstanding surface. A number of the contributors to this volume have remarked on the fact that staff members are likely to feel threatened by what is perceived as an undesirable intrusion on their privacy and security by an outsider. It is important for the consultant to actively engage the cooperation of staff members and allay their fears if the consultation is to proceed successfully. It is extremely important to understand the needs of the consultee, and a "consultee needs assessment," while possibly lengthening the initial preprogram stage, helps ensure that subsequent programs are more relevant and will have greater impact.

The problem-solving phase comprises the major issue of consultation. Alternative solutions are outlined, and a program of constructive action is devised. The termination phase is reached by mutual agreement and should include some evaluation component with which to assess the degree to which various goals have been achieved.

THE VALUE OF CONSULTATION

Factors Affecting Outcome

Successful consultation depends on a variety of factors, only some of which may be considered objective. The most successful programs are those that have been perceived by the client as relevant. To assure relevance, the consultant and client need to work closely together, to establish good lines of communication, to enlist as broad a basis of support and participation among the client's employees as possible, and to gather feedback at various stages during the consultation process so that immediate modifications can be incorporated as the need for them arises.

From the outset the consultant's role must be clearly stated, and expectations should be realistic. The consultant should feel supported by the agency administration and should expect cooperation on all reasonable requests. Concurrently, the client should feel confidence in the consultant, and an effort must be made so that the significance of all consultant demands is understood.

Jacoby (1974) has detailed a cogent set of guidelines for the consultant. Most important, and a point on which all contributors to this volume agree, is that expectations on the part of the client should be realistic. To this end, the consultant should never promise more than can be delivered. In fact, Jacoby (1974) recommends delivering a little more than promised. It is important here to recognize one's own limitations as a consultant while at the same time not undervaluing oneself and one's time. The focus should be on what the consultant can do for the client. Project reports should be readily accessible in terms of both length and readability. An effort must be made to realistically anticipate all costs; the client has a right not to be saddled with unexpectedly high costs once the program is underway. In a similar vein, Jacoby (1974) strongly recommends informing the client of "bad news" as soon as it is discovered; nothing is gained in the long run from the unrealistic expectations generated by an inadequately informed client.

Unfortunately, little systematic research has been done on the relationship between various factors in the process of consultation and the client's perception of outcome. (The recommendations detailed in this section have necessarily been drawn largely from the subjective impressions of individuals actively engaged in consulting work; be aware that they have the compelling force of all observations that appear to be logical.) This area strongly deserves future attention, and a number of investigators are beginning to articulate potentially fruitful channels for research. Bindman (1966) recommends that research on consultation could most productively focus on several areas: (1) consultant behaviors (what is done and how does it relate to outcome?); (2) consultee behaviors (what are their attitudes and motivations?); and (3) organizational and situational variables affecting outcome. The very scope of these recommended areas indicates how little empirical knowledge exists with respect to consultation.

Training to Be a "Good" Consultant

The oldest model of consultation is one in which one professional is asked by another professional to give an expert opinion (Bindman, 1966). This model often predominates the clinical psychologist consultant—client interaction, especially within the mental health professions. However, clinical psychologists are now beginning to be asked for their expert opinions in areas traditionally, considered to fall within the realm of psychiatry. For instance, psychologists are more frequently being called as expert witnesses in court to give testimony with respect to such questions as criminal responsibility, competence to stand trial, capacity to manage one's own affairs, child custody, and mental status. The psychologist can usually feel quite comfortable with having the skill and ability to meet the need for this service. On the other hand, within government and industrial sectors consultation is less likely to relate so exclusively to giving expert opinion. In these cases, consultation involves advice and guidance to "help insure [that] human resources are adequate to achieve company goals *and* that these resources are properly developed and deployed and appropriately utilized" (Sashkin & Kunin, this volume [emphasis added]). To this end the consultant may become involved in designing programs, running employee groups, reorganizing departments, and evaluating outcome information. Similarly, all three types of service detailed earlier are called into play by psychologists who are breaking new professional ground in their roles as consultants to correctional institutions. Here, specifically, the consultant may be requested to investigate the adequacy of inmate service delivery, evaluate the need for and initiate new programs for inmates (e.g., vocational and educational programs), and develop useful diagnostic and classification instruments as well as evaluate a variety of institutional procedures. The need for expertise in each of these areas will vary with the unique requirements of each new client. The psychological consultant may be only partially prepared to meet the needs of these clients by the more traditional academic training he has received in graduate school. Certainly he is likely to be adequately prepared to provide diagnostic and testing expertise, but in the wider areas of developing alternative programs, be they for an industrial client or for a correctional institution, the psychological consultant is often placed at a distinct disadvantage by his lack of experience.

A number of observers have addressed the issue of training the psychological consultant. Formal exposure to the methods and techniques of consultation, perhaps by means of the case method and practicum training, would be ideal. However, in the absence of such structured opportunities the psychology graduate student may still develop a strong background for developing good consultant techniques, especially in light of the student's purported conversance with the dynamics of interpersonal situations. Specific recommendations include courses in personality and psychodynamics, experience in psychotherapy, training in diagnostic appraisal, some experience in educational methods, and a knowledge of social psychology, administration principles, and the organization of community resources (Bindman, 1966). Additionally it is likely that the psychological consultant will have to draw on well-developed skills in selecting and developing survey instruments at some point in his consulting career.

These recommendations are fairly general and should serve the psychological consultant well in any chosen field. However, more specific skills and familiarity with professional principles and jargon may be required in some areas, notably business and industry. For instance, Sashkin and Kunin (this volume) recommend as a requirement for such practice a doctoral degree in industrial-organizational psychology with formal training in personnel selection and assessment. Practical orientation in courses offered by a business school will be invaluable to the consultant to business. Sashkin and Kunin's advice that one should adapt one's skills to the client's needs rather than adapting client needs to one's own discipline is enormously valuable whatever one's chosen arena. Beyond these rather general principles, each consultant will find no substitute for actual experience (albeit trial and error at times). Information such as that contained in the present volume should provide some additional guidance by those who are currently consulting in the areas of education, government, industry, and criminal justice.

EXPANDING OPPORTUNITIES FOR THE PSYCHOLOGICAL CONSULTANT

As noted earlier, psychologists are being asked to consult to an ever-increasing variety of institutions and individuals. Some of these areas are fairly traditional, and the format of consultation is well established. Other areas represent new opportunities for psychologists, and the delineation of their consultant roles is commensurately less clear. Only a brief overview of the opportunities for consultation in the fields of business, government, public health, education, and criminal justice will be presented here; the reader is referred to the more detailed discussions offered by the various contributors to this volume for a more comprehensive treatment.

Community Consultation

One role into which psychologists have increasingly found themselves thrust, either by choice or by default, is that of mental health consultant to an entire community. This may represent an active and exciting choice on the part of those working as federal and regional consultants for such governmental agencies as the National Institute of Mental Health. On the other hand, it may represent an anxiety-inducing situation for those who, understandably, feel overwhelmed to find themselves unexpectedly the only professional with any training in mental health matters in a given geographic region. In either case the psychological consultant is asked to give advice to such diverse professionals as public health physicians, clergy, judges, welfare workers, teachers, police officers, and members of community planning boards. Such psychologists have aptly been called by Libo (1966) '' 'generalists'—as general practitioners in human welfare services'' (p. 530).

As a community consultant, the psychologist will deal with an entire network of community agencies. Often he will be forced to develop alternatives to the traditional resources in dealing with an individual's problems, particularly in the more rural areas of the country. This may also involve coordinating planning between existing community organizations and case consultation to various agencies and practitioners as well as in-service training to these same agencies. Some of the consultant's work will, of course, require the traditional psychological skills. At the same time, as Libo (1966) has pointed out, in order to establish high visibility as a resource person, other personal characteristics will be essential. Personal and social skills are a must in community work. The community consultant, to a far greater degree than the traditional private practitioner, should be outgoing, possess a high energy level, have a broad range of interests, and, perhaps most importantly, possess substantial patience to deal with people as they are (Libo, 1966). The opportunity to expedite interagency communication, referrals, and coordination of services, to provide case consultation and direct clinical services, to conduct educational and training programs, and to organize and expand mental health—related facilities may appeal to some psychologists who are exploring the opportunities for consulting work. For the psychologist seeking a broadly based career with relatively little structure and a great deal of autonomy, such a position may provide tremendous excitement and challenge.

Mental Health Consultation with Groups

Another opportunity exists to reach a large number of people while at the same time limiting one's obligations to fit more closely the skills acquired in traditional psychology training. As a group consultant, the psychologist will assist key professionals within a community to carry out their primary responsibilities. The group method allows the consultant to reach a large number of professionals within a limited time while simultaneously using group members' affective involvement with their work problems to distinct advantage. While consultation with groups resembles both group supervision and seminar teaching, it differs from therapy in that the content focus is not on the personal problems but the work problems of the individual members (Altrocchi, Spielberger, & Eisdorfer, 1965). These work problems are likely to be shared by at least several group members, and general group theory suggests that peer influence can be aroused and channeled in this situation to generate productive solutions. The consultant's primary goal will be to help the group develop solutions on their own to common work problems. The consultant acts as a catalyst to help clarify consultee attitudes (Altrocchi et al., 1965). Opportunities for such consulting positions are likely to exist in numerous communities and should appeal to the psychologist who enjoys working with groups and finds the group process an exciting and productive means of effecting change.

Consultation to Schools

Dorr (this volume) compellingly argues the importance to our educational system of consulting. It is not surprising that this area has experienced considerable growth in the past decade in the number of psychological consultants. This area is certainly not a new one for psychological consultants; however, while recognizing the attractiveness of educational consultation, Dorr also realistically analyzes the forces leading to the dissatisfaction and frustration experienced by many psychologists who have chosen this particular area. Noting that there is likely to be some conflict between the goals of the consultant as psychologist and the teacher as client, Dorr carefully outlines some of the barriers a psychological consultant may expect to encounter in trying to implement his proposals. The consultant needs to be especially sensitive to the demand factors affecting school systems, notably what the public expects the systems to accomplish. It should appear obvious that teachers are not evaluated with respect to the mental health of their pupils, but this fact is often unwittingly overlooked by the psychological consultant who feels his valuable proposals for change have been ignored. The consultant needs to realize that he is operating within an arena where various constituencies are represented and that misconceptions may frequently stall the best-guided efforts. Dorr's chapter should provide valuable information and advice for the psychologist interested in or currently pursuing a career consulting within the educational system.

Consultants in the Corrections System

Similarly, Gendreau and Andrews (this volume) have opened up discussion on a new field of consulting that is increasingly drawing psychologists concerned about the status of our criminal justice system. The expansion of client services in the corrections system that occurred throughout the 1960s and into the 1970s in attempting to shift the focus to rehabilitation rather than punishment has lead to the increased use of psychologists particularly in service delivery. Psychological consultation to correctional institutions is still controversial, with as much success reported as failure. As Gendreau and Andrews point out, one of the major issues in consultation of this type is the continued maintenance and growth of a program after the consultants leave. To this end they discuss the importance of involving insitutional staff in various phases of the consultation process.

Of perhaps equal importance to the success of the consultation endeavor is the unfortunate but pervasive lack of knowledge on the part of psychologists just entering the prison system as to what really works in corrections. Gendreau and Andrews point out that while much is gained via trial and error, the opportunities that exist for using traditional psychological skills, for learning, and for effecting social change are perhaps unparalleled. Their detailed advice to the psychologist interested in consulting to correctional institutions is noteworthy.

Consultation to the Courts and to Police

Psychologists are increasingly being asked to consult both to the courts and to police departments. In both cases they must draw predominantly on clinical skills. As noted earlier, psychologists are more frequently than in the past being asked to give expert testimony on such issues as criminal responsibility, competency to stand trial or to manage one's own affairs, child custody, test validity, and mental status. Kaslow (this volume) eloquently and compellingly argues in favor of the psychologist's responsibility to offer his clinical input to the judicial system. As she notes, who is better qualified to assess an individual's needs than the psychologist? However, the consultant's role does not end in the witness chair. Kaslow strongly suggests an important place exists for psychologists in research and program evaluation to aid judges in understanding the relationship between their decisions and eventual outcomes as well as in influencing mental health legislation. Her chapter also suggests possibilities and provides extremely useful information to the psychologist interested in consulting to the criminal justice system.

Similarly, the chapter by Fenster and Schlossberg on consultation to police departments outlines a wide range of services that the psychologist can provide. While many of these services relate directly to clinical skills, such as counseling police personnel and their families, others have the appeal of being potentially dramatic and exciting, such as working in hostage situations. The authors also note the frustration inherent in an attempt to effect change within any bureaucracy. Their thoughts highlight an area of increasing need for psychological consultation, one that is often overlooked by the novice consultant.

Consultation to Government and Industry

These fields are those traditionally thought of when consultation is mentioned. Both offer well-established opportunities for full- or part-time consultation work. Consultants may remain academically based while engaging in part-time work on short-range projects or advisory committees. In industry, particularly, there may be a strong research element to the consultant's activities in human engineering, aptitude and personality testing, altering employee attitudes and motivations, and group dynamics. Considerable effort may be directed at job design and at making necessary work more meaningful for the employee. For psychologists with strong interests in the functioning of business, the chapter by Sashkin and Kunin on consulting to industry may provide the information necessary to initiate a search for such contacts.

Similarly, the chapter by Cook and Buccino on government consultation is full of practical and detailed advice. The consultant to government may operate as an individual giving expert advice, as a member of an advisory committee, or as a member of a contract firm writing proposals or managing grant contracts. Cook and Buccino indicate a growing opportunity for psychological consultants in the government with the trend toward an increased Federal role in all areas of life concomitant with increased need for technical skills in order to keep up with expanded service delivery.

REFERENCES

Altrocchi, J., Spielberger, C. D., & Eisdorfer, C. Mental health consultation with groups. *Community Mental Health Journal*, 1965, *1*, 127–134.

Bindman, A. J. The clinical psychologist as a mental health consultant. *Progress in clinical psychology*. New York: Grune & Stratton, 1966.

Burke, R. J. Psychologists consult with organizations: Alternative strategies of involvement. *The Canadian Psychologist*, 1971, *12*, 482–497.

Jacoby, J. The roles, values and training of a consultant. Paper No. 141. *Purdue Papers in Consumer Psychology*. Purdue University, 1974.

Libo, L. M. Multiple functions for psychologists in community consultation. *American Psychologist*, 1966, *21*, 530–534.

Pearl, A. The psychological consultant as change agent. *Professional Psychology*, 1974, *5*, 292–298.

Smith, T. S., & Sorenson, J. E. *Integrated management information systems for community mental health centers*. Rockville, Md.: NIMH, 1974.

Darwin Dorr

2

Psychological Consulting in the Schools

Most youngsters attend school 9 months a year for at least 6 hours a day. For years children have spent more time in their schools than they did with their fathers; now, as more and more women begin to work full-time jobs, children spend more time with their teachers than they do with their mothers. Epidemiologic studies have shown that a large minority of these school children manifest some form of educational, behavioral, or emotional maladjustment (Cowen, Zax, Izzo, & Trost, 1966; Glidewell & Swallow, 1969; Kellam & Schiff, 1967). Unchecked, such problems often lead to the development of major mental and/or behavioral maladaptation, which takes a massive toll economically (Dorr, 1972) and in terms of personal suffering.

Viewing these circumstances, the authors of *Action for Mental Health* (1961) published by the Joint Commission on Mental Health offered the following observations regarding schools:

Here, then, is a ready-made setting with the potentiality for directing, reinforcing, or correcting mental health. The school may not only guide, strengthen, or even treat the mental health of the pupil, but also through the role of the pupil as a family member seek means of improving home situations for the sake of all members of the family (p. 124).

It is reasonable, perhaps mandatory, to bring the knowledge of many disciplines to the process of education in order to prevent the development of emotional disorders and, ideally, to make a positive contribution toward a student's development of personal growth that will lead to a higher realization of human potential in adulthood. The recognition of the problems and potentialities of school systems has led in recent years to a dramatic increase in the involvement of psychologists in schools, particularly in the role of consultant.

Psychologists can potentially make a significant contribution to the process of education. First, many psychologists are well trained in developmental psychology, an area directly relevant to cognitive training as well as to behavioral management of children. Furthermore, many psychologists are trained in mental health interventions and are able to recognize and treat children and advise educators regarding the most effective and therapeutic way of handling such emotional and behavioral problems in children. The contributions of psychologists to educational tests and measurement are well documented. Finally, in recent years psychologists, particularly those with a community and/or social psychological orientation, have become knowledgeable in the area of systems and organizations, a knowledge that can be helpful in working toward a positive outcome for children caught in the inner workings of the school's organizational machinery.

Despite their potential to help, psychologists who attempt to consult in schools often fail miserably. Psychological consultation in the schools is an extremely difficult and frustrating enterprise largely because of the special characteristics of the target system. Schools tend to be powerful, committed to a status quo, conservative, cautious, and sometimes reactionary. By necessity schools reflect the culture of the citizens whose taxes support them, rendering schools, like our society, variable and complex. Schools' "personalities" vary with geographical location, local and state political sentiments, personal characteristics of principal and teachers, and the dominant problems of the children. All of these factors contribute to the development of a matrix, and sometimes a maze, of forces, political and personal in nature, that have the potential to render the psychological consultant's well-intended efforts meaningless or worse. Psychologists who fail as consultants in the schools are usually defeated not by lack of fundamental knowledge in the area of psychology, or, for that matter, by lack of knowledge of the consultation process; rather, they fail usually because they lack understanding of ways to effectively deal with the curious complexities of modern American school systems.

One would expect that psychologists trained to understand and deal with the complexities of human behavior would be very effective in school systems, yet psychologists as a group tend to focus on individual patients or clients. As a result, many psychologists set aside their scientifically professional point of view when dealing with social systems, often regressing to a naively moralistic point of view in castigating "the system" as a villainous monster that is, at best, an ineffective baby-sitting service and, at worst, an ill-intended, malevolent perpetrator of outrageous atrocities upon children. Some psychologists advocate the total destruction and remaking of our public school systems.

Unfortunately, even if such anarchistic fantasies could be made to come true, I know of no data that make me confident that we have the knowledge and understanding to rebuild a school system to conform to utopian dreams. It is fruitless to waste energy debating whether schools are good or bad; it is more productive to begin by accepting the realities of our schools. In the final analysis, schools are merely aggregates of human beings, with all of their frailties, arrogance, and foolishness. It is obvious that the system is imperfect and, like the individual, likely to resist change even if such change were for the best. In my view the mission of the psychological consultant is to help persons within the schools do their job more effectively and to improve their coordinated efforts (their system) when and where such improvement is necessary and/or possible.

This chapter offers suggestions that will help consultants achieve positive ends in their endeavors in the schools. The majority of my discussion is intended to sensitize consultants to the special characteristics and features of the system of schools and educators. My metapurpose is to help psychologists become as insightful, professional, and understanding with regard to school systems as they are with their individual patients and clients. To this end, I will first examine the school system in relation to the matrix of other social helping institutions. Following this, I will attempt to paint a picture of the social anatomy of schools, focusing on both the internal and external forces that impinge upon, shape, and maintain the system. Preentry factors are then considered, followed by a discussion of psychologist—educator communication and expectancy problems. The special dangers that face the psychological consultant in the schools are reviewed. Finally, I will summarize examples of various exemplary approaches to consultation in the schools, including consulting from a particular personality theory, consulting from a particular interventive stance, and consulting from a system's analysis point of view.

UNDERSTANDING SCHOOL SYSTEMS

The School's Place Among Helping Institutions

It will be helpful to view schools from a broad social perspective. Penetrating reviews of social factors influencing schools have been written by Trickett, Kelly, and Todd (1972), Sarason (1971), and Bower (1972). Bower viewed schools as one of several "humanizing institutions" created by human beings to socialize their own kind. Bower divided these institutions into primary, secondary, and tertiary groups. Tertiary humanizing institutions, abbreviated ICE (illness correctional endeavors), available to those people with major problems, consist of state and federal prisons, state and mental hospitals, and other 24-hour care facilities that provide a maximum of care and a minimum of freedom. The secondary group, AID (ailing—in difficulty) institutions, includes physicians and hospitals, attorneys and courts of law, varieties of social agencies, clinics, county jails, homes for children, special schools and programs, counsellors, and others. The purpose of these institutions is to restore health, economic independence, and social or emotional competence.

The primary institutions, called KISS institutions (key integrative social systems), include (1) the health-enhancing agencies, especially those responsible for the health of pregnant women, (2) the family, (3) informal peer groups, including informal and formal recreation and play institutions, and (4) the school. Bower pointed out that while society does not expect that every child will receive adequate prenatal care or live in a happy home, it does expect that the school will be successful with every child; i.e., the school is supposed to be successful even when the other KISS institutions are inadequate or ineffectual. Hence in comparison to other major humanizing institutions the demands on schools are great.

Demand Factors Influencing Schools

Society extends little sympathy to the school that fails to humanize. The school's part in the humanization enterprise is to educate youngsters, but as we begin attempts to implement this broad, misty aim, we encounter difficulties. Most people have their own versions of what the schools should be doing; the consultant needs to be aware of these expectations. For example, one could argue that the "real" primary goal of schools is to make jobs and keep children off the streets. While it is cynical, this claim has some valid basis; the consultant can profit from keeping it in mind.

Another goal is the teaching of basic subject matter, particularly the "3 R's." While many readers will argue that there is much more to education than this, one must remember that educators, like so many people, feel that the first job of schools is to help children acquire basic facility in dealing with the major communicative symbols of their culture. Additionally, the consultant should be aware that in the final analysis, when teachers are evaluated the major metric is the degree to which their children have mastered these basic factors. Teachers are rarely evaluated on the level of mental health among their children. In view of this, it is not surprising that external forces that attempt to interfere with progress toward this particular, fundamental goal will often be met with stout resistance.

While few people would disagree that schools should teach basics, many press toward a richer and more humanistic educational system, which has led to enormous pressures on educators from all sides. For example, musicians feel that more music education will sensitize youngsters to a world of music beyond what they hear on their radios and perhaps teach them some musical skills that they can use for recreational purposes and self-development for years to come. Artists mount similar campaigns. Gym teachers bemoan the physical decline of Americans and press for innovative and universal physical education programs. Home economists and industrial arts teachers rightfully point out that practical life skills are necessary and on a decline, and they push for more training in these areas. So it goes for librarians.

Concerns for children's special problems have dramatically increased the number of special helpers—we have counsellors, social workers, speech therapists, and special teachers for EMRs, TMRs, deaf children, emotionally disturbed children, intellectually gifted children, and disadvantaged children, and there are school nurses, physicians, and audiologists, as well as helping teachers, resource teachers, perceptual disorder specialists, and a host of other usually well-trained and well-intended persons. All provide many helpful services for children, but they put enormous demands on "the system" to alter itself to be more sensitive to the special needs of their diverse approaches.

There are also demands made on the school by the community. Schools must deal with many special-interest groups, parents, and civic leaders. Schools are often "political footballs." One current debate involves the matter of social promotion and automatic high school diploma merely for attendance. Sex education is commonly a major issue of concern, as is religious (and for that matter political) education. Finally, for various reasons our schools today have become excellent places for youngsters to learn about drugs, alcohol, and other sociopathic problems, and the school is expected to deal with all of these social ills.

In view of the number and power of the forces impinging on it, what is the school to do? It must be sensitive to these forces because it is a tax-supported institution and must respond to the taxpayers. On the other hand, the school cannot be all things to all people—this is impossible because of limited manpower and because the school has finite resources, namely, the moneys (from taxes) that pay people's salaries. Hence the school must develop a defensive posture that will allow it to continue its daily work and that usually appears as the institutional barriers that psychologists and others often find incredibly frustrating. However, it is helpful to realize that organizations, like people, need a certain number of barriers to protect themselves against extraneous forces, which may foster positive feedback to the system, usually resulting in system disruption. While system disruption is usually necessary for positive change, a system that is constantly disrupted simply cannot function very effectively. A combination of or balance between status quo and change is needed if the system is to evolve in an orderly and constructive manner.

The psychologist hoping for longevity as a school consultant must be aware that he or she is in actuality only a tiny factor in the universe of vectors and countervectors that impinge upon the school system. The system has a right to evaluate and perhaps shun the consultant's efforts, and he or she must realize that this defensive posture sometimes arises for other reasons than ignorance. On the other hand, as part of the school's ecologic network the psychologist has a perfect right to attempt to effect positive feedback to the school system in hopes of improving system functioning and services for children.

PREENTRY FACTORS TO CONSIDER BEFORE CONSULTING IN THE SCHOOLS

Having reviewed some socioecologic forces, we now turn to some more practical matters. A first step in consulting is to determine whether or not to get involved with a school in the first place. Many problems in consultation occur because the consultant contract is not clearly thought out by either the consultee or the consultant. The results may be hurt feelings and wasted time and money. Cherniss (1976) discussed some of these issues at length. The first question Cherniss asked is, "Should one provide consultation in this situation?" He points out that there are always alternatives to consultation; these should always be understood by the consultant and the consultee. Interestingly, one of the major functions of the consultant is to open up the consultee to alternative solutions. Hence it seems that the best place to start focusing on alternatives is at the preentry stage. Cherniss provides an example in which he participated in a meeting of a school consultation project. A consultant in the school had been consulting primarily with a rather high-placed school administrator; this seemed logical, but the sessions were unproductive. No one had asked the question, "Why should we provide consultation to this person?" When the question finally was asked, there was some confusion and embarrassment, and it was finally decided that this person was the consultee because he had high status in the system. Of course, high status does not necessarily make the individual the most likely consultee. Cherniss cites guidelines for systematically deciding whether or not to consult in a given setting. Major issues are (1) the relationship between the consultant's system; (2) the congruence between the consultant's own values and those of the consultee; (3) consultee characteristics (e.g., "Are these individuals that I can work with and that I can help?"); and (4) the consultant's place in the social milieu of the consultee's system.

The second major question Cherniss asks is, "Whose interest will the consultant serve? Who are the [constituents]?" There will be, particularly in schools, diverse interest groups. Cherniss cites Waller (1967), who argued that in the classroom, students and teachers often represent different and antagonistic interests. While it is tempting to say that the interests of all parties are being served by consulting, this is not necessarily true and will not necessarily be perceived as such by the various constituencies.

A final question is, "What will be the primary focus of the consultation?" In my experience, failure to evaluate this question and to reevaluate it at significant times often leads to confusion. Will the consultant focus on organization, structure, and process, or on technology (e.g., skills, techniques, and processes required to perform particular tasks), on the mental health of individuals, or on group or organizational environment?

It is best to consider these issues as thoroughly as possible prior to entering the system and to reconsider them in the early phases of the consultation, continuing to clarify the relationship between consultee and consultant and modeling a way of analytically examining purpose and function that will serve as a good model for problem solving later on in the consultant relationship.

PSYCHOLOGISTS versus EDUCATORS

We have seen that many characters play a part in the social drama within and between schools, yet from our view the most important communications take place between educator and psychologist. While the goal is a harmonious enlightening and helpful dialogue between two willing and enthusiastic professionals of different stripes, their differences can often get in the way. In this section some problems in educator-psychologist communication will be discussed. Since communication problems are often the result of incompatible perceptions and expectations, we will focus on the way these two groups view each other and themselves.

Educators' Views of Psychologists

Virtually everyone in the school will be forming an impression of the consultant entering the school, and these impressions may often be at odds with the consultant's self-image. The psychologist in the schools may be viewed variously as a socialistic meddler, a mind reader, a psychotherapist, a psychoanalyst, a threat, a savior, and a tester. Unfortunately, the expectancies that teachers hold for psychologists are not always matched by the expectancies and goals of the psychologist. For example, Roberts (1970) surveyed psychologists and teachers regarding the role of the psychologist in seven different areas—psychometry, diagnostics, consultation, mental hygiene, research, therapy, and educational programming. Roberts reached the following conclusions:

1. There is considerable diversity in the perceptions and evaluations by the teacher and the psychologist of the functions actually performed by the school psychologist.
2. Psychologists and teachers differ considerably in their reports of how the psychologist distributes his time and emphasis.
3. There is great diversity of opinion as to the functions of the psychologist under desired or more ideal circumstances.
4. Psychologists report that they "should be" involved more than they are in most types of activities (except for the psychometrician roles, which they think are overemphasized).

Sometimes these misperceptions are humorous. For example, when I consult in a school I usually try to eat in the school cafeteria, both because it is convenient and because it gives me an opportunity to be with children and to get a sense of the school. While in the lunch line I have often heard the kitchen workers remark that they had better not say too much when the "head-shrinker" is in the lunch line or lest their minds be read. However, communication-perception difficulties are often more serious. A few years ago some colleagues and I were attempting to develop a small mental health program in an elementary school. The program combined consultation with the use of aides to work with youngsters who were having some adjustive difficulties. One community person was adamantly against the project because she felt that we were out to "psychoanalyze" the children. While she did not understand what we were doing, she "knew" that whatever it was, it was decidedly a bad thing. She protested vigorously in the school board meeting when funding for our project was being discussed. The school board passed the project, at which point this person cried out, "God help our children," and hysterically collapsed in her chair. She had a decidedly different perception of what we would be doing than we had ourselves.

Educators' Views of Educators

The consultant ought to be sensitive to educators' self-perceptions, since there can be misconceptions that can lead to difficulties. Parker (1962) and Berlin (1956) observed in their consultation practices several beliefs that can be counterproductive, particularly in achieving mental health goals in the classroom. Berlin noted that in the presence of the consultant many teachers were afraid to show anger toward their children, even when it was justified. I have experienced many examples of this in my own consulting experiences. For example, on one occasion in an elementary school a certain youngster was, as usual, out of line and creating a disturbance. The principal, a talented and warmhearted woman, scolded him for his shenanigans and insisted that he get back in line and behave like the other children. I was standing behind her when this occurred. She turned to me with a glare and rather sarcastically said, "I suppose that I've now destroyed his poor little psyche," and stomped off. I had not said a word and indeed was in support of her action, but apparently she had some feelings about teachers showing anger toward children.

Another misconception that Berlin found in teachers is that they believe that they must be "fond" of all their pupils, yet children are very perceptive and can usually see through artificial shows of affection in a teacher who basically does not care much for them.

Parker (1962), surveying nursery school teachers, found that they sometimes hold three somewhat different artificial beliefs: (1) If you understand a problem, you should be able to solve it. (Many psychologists believe this, too.) (2) A really good teacher never dislikes a child. (3) A prime goal of nursery school is to help the child become integrated in a group. While there is some degree of truth in each of these, it is obviously unrealistic to believe that these principles are always true.

Psychologists' Views of Educators

Psychologists tend to be arrogant about their own profession, particularly in relation to the profession of education. Education is often seen as a low-status endeavor. Iscoe commented on this arrogance in his Special Award Presentation at the APA convention in 1976. In an article based on this presentation (1977), he reminds us that in terms of power to deal with children we have little to be arrogant about. Educators, not psychologists, have the children, the schools, the money, and the political clout. Additionally, Iscoe urges psychologists to be more open-minded regarding teachers and more willing to engage in a give-and-take relationship.

It is fairly easy for the psychologist to become intolerant of teachers who become angry or frustrated or intolerant of the children they are dealing with, yet the psychologist, as many teachers point out, may have never taught in the regular classroom. Teachers have needs, as do other individuals, and, being human beings, most teachers easily experience anger, frustration, love, compassion, spite, jealousy, and the whole range of human emotions. Teaching is a very difficult and demanding task, and it is not surprising that teachers sometimes lose their tempers. However, I think that most teachers go into teaching because of a basic love for children and a desire to be loved in return.

An example from the history of the Primary Mental Health Project in Rochester, N. Y. (Cowen, Trost, Lorion, Dorr, Izzo, & Isaacson, 1975) makes this dramatically clear. When the Project first began to employ child aides, the aides were placed in the classroom. As the months went by it became clear that there was a great deal of resistance from the teachers regarding the child aides, which caused considerable tension until our psychoanalytic consultant pointed out that most persons go into teaching because of a love for children and a desire to be loved by them in return. The aides were apparently getting all of the love and affection from the children, since they were perceived as the "warm mommas," and the teachers bore the burden of the instructional work and disciplinary tasks. We had, in effect, short-circuited the source of the teachers' major reinforcement, which made them justifiably resentful. This led to a necessary change in the relationships among aide, children, and teacher. If most of these teachers did not basically feel some tenderness toward children, they probably would not have been bothered by the role that the aides had usurped.

Ogden Lindsley (1972) forcefully points out the need to be realistic and perceptive regarding our views of teachers. He reminds us that the education profession is massive, and because of its size educators reflect roughly the distribution of competence, compassion, sensitivity, and other human qualities that are exhibited in the general population. There are dull teachers, average teachers, and brilliant teachers. There are cruel teachers and kind teachers. Psychologists tend to have a stereotypic view of teachers, which often leads to difficulties in communication. Each teacher must be evaluated in terms of his or her own individual competencies and talents. This is particularly true with regard to teachers' knowledge of mental health principles—some are incredibly naive and resistant to mental health principles, and others are outstanding psychologists.

Another bias that psychologists often have is that "brightness" is "goodness." This prejudice, acquired from years in academe, can be decidedly inappropriate in the school setting. In my own experience, I have known some extremely bright individuals who were very poor teachers and I have known some teachers who were rather dull intellectually but who were excellent at their job, being gifted in other ways such as warmth, compassion, and sensitivity.

COUNTERTRANSFERENCE PROBLEMS OF THE CONSULTANT

A major aspect of psychotherapeutic training is the development of self-protective strategies that will shield the therapist from harmful emotional entanglements with the patient. The longer one practices the art of psychotherapy, the more one recognizes the importance of this aspect of training. Unfortunately, in preparation for the consultant role there is almost no emphasis placed on a similar effort to protect the consultant from his own emotionality when dealing with systems, yet this preparation and training is particularly helpful when dealing with school systems. A personal example will illustrate this.

The incident occurred during my first year of consulting in the schools (1964). The date is important because of social forces active at that time. The event took place in an elementary school in a white, blue-collar, rural-suburban area in the Northeast. One of the upper grade teachers had a black youngster that he claimed was a troublemaker. Indeed, the child did have a long history of predelinquent- and delinquent-type behavior and was at that time separated by law from his parents because he bordered on being incorrigible and because he had a long history of being subjected to severe child abuse. Obviously such misguided attempts at discipline only made the boy worse.

In my opinion, the boy was responding to school and was forming a therapeutic relationship with one of the special teachers. The classroom teacher, however, complained repeatedly about this youngster and took his complaints to the principal. The principal strongly believed in standing up for his teachers. Finally, a crisis erupted when the youngsters were walking in a line to a group activity. There was an altercation between the boy and the teacher in which the child struck out at the teacher and the teacher subdued the youngster. Over my objections, the principal then went to higher school officials and demanded that the child be removed from the school. Because of the structure of the laws, the child could not remain in his foster home placement if he did not attend school, and the only alternative was to send him to the state hospital.

This was a considerable blow to me because I had invested time and care in the youngster and was hoping that we might effect some therapeutic change before he went on to junior high school. I was not confident that the outcome would be in the best interest of the youngster.

Later, disappointment changed to anger. I was involved in a social event some months later that included the boy's ex-teacher, and we found ourselves in the same car en route to the party. We happened to drive through a section of town that was largely black, and he expressed his revulsion over being in this part of town. Later, after consuming several beers, he proudly told me that the black youngster had actually been no real trouble in his class; rather the youngster did not participate very actively in the work, and the teacher had decided he was not going to let the boy get away with this. The teacher then went on to explain how he intentionally teased and badgered the boy into the altercation in the hallway, and when the boy lashed out in anger the teacher had the opportunity to physically attack him with impunity. He explained how he tripped the boy and then performed a knee drop into the boy's stomach "to teach that black S.O.B. a lesson."

Many persons reading this chapter will have had a similar experience or will have one sometime in the future. This kind of incident is not uncommon in school systems. How does the consultant deal with these issues? In my opinion, it would be an error to prepare the consultant to be unaffected by such social violence. There is a place for righteous indignation, social reform, and radical system change, yet there are many frustrated "good Samaritans" who have become so embittered with their helping experiences that they merely drop out, e.g., *Up the Down Staircase* (Kaufman, 1964). Dropping out is understandable, but it does nothing for the children we came to help in the first place.

How could I have been more effective in dealing with the situation I encountered? We will never know whether there actually was a better way to deal with the situation, but upon reflection I can identify some counter-transference forces that perhaps limited my degree of effectiveness. Major factors were (1) my attitude toward schools, (2) my attitude toward myself, (3) my view of the youngster, including his race, and (4) my attitude toward the teacher and principal. Did I have lingering resentments toward schools? Let us examine each factor in turn.

Susan Gray (a pioneer in the area of school psychology) points out in her textbook of school psychology (1963) that psychologists entering school systems would be advised to examine their feelings and attitudes toward school systems based on their own experiences as pupils. Lingering resentments can only lead to fantasies of revenge that are counterproductive and inappropriate. What about my attitude toward myself? While I would not then publicly admit to it, having been a pupil many, many years, it was relatively easy to lapse into what the transactional analysts call the "child state" of ego. In the child state feelings of helplessness and deference may lead to feelings of anger, resentment, and perceptions of teachers and administrators as the "them" that we never trusted in junior high school. Such a stance is obviously counterproductive. The third factor was my view of the youngster, particularly his race. As noted, this episode occurred during the emotional early stages of the integration movement. As I look back, I think I flew to this youngster's defense fully oblivious to the fact that he could be extremely disruptive. Had I been more aware of these feelings and perhaps more realistic with regard to the boy, I would have been able to respond to the teacher's needs and cries for help more effectively, which, perhaps, might have headed off his violent response to his frustrations.

The fourth factor was my attitude toward the teacher and the principal. Obviously, these attitudes were intertwined with the factors noted above.

Because I became angry with the teacher and principal, I was insensitive to their needs. The teacher needed to feel in control of his classroom. He was effective with the youngsters under his care. Furthermore, it was not necessarily my job as a consultant to change this man's biases but rather to bring him to respond more fairly with regard to the youngsters against whom he was biased. Finally, while it is true that the principal was shortsighted and insensitive to all of the factors that transpired, he was intent on doing a good job in the school system. He had become principal when the school was an administrative disaster area, and he had attempted to establish some structure and support for the teachers who previously had felt very unsupported. Thus he probably saw my efforts to support the youngster as directly threatening his goals, which were to raise the morale of the faculty in his school through his support of them.

All of the above is speculation; I do not know if proper consideration of these factors would have led me to be more effective in the situation. However, I feel that there has been relatively little attention given to these "countertransference issues" in the process of consultation. In my experience, they are very real, very powerful, and sometimes very destructive.

SOME MODELS OF SCHOOL CONSULTATION

To this point we have focused primarily on system and communication factors within the schools in order to sensitize the reader to the kinds of forces that will help or hinder the consultant's efforts. We will now examine some exemplary models of consultation. The purpose of this review is to demonstrate that while there are many common elements in school consultation, there is also considerable room for variation in theoretical orientation and interventive stance. For example, some consultants find special merit in a particular personality or behavioral theory; as a result their consultive interventions tend to emphasize certain factors over others. Three examples will be reviewed to illustrate this orientation—consulting from traditional psychoanalytic, Adlerian, and behavioral points of view.

Other consultants prefer to consult from a particular preventive stance. While most school consultation is of the case-centered variety and therefore generally some form of tertiary prevention, some consultants attempt to adopt a secondary or even primary preventive orientation. Examples of each of these last two will be reviewed.

Finally, many consultants are now advocating a more or less "systems" point of view, which is, in part, a special type of primary prevention. Examples of this approach will be reviewed briefly.

Consulting from a Psychodynamic Point of View

In *The Mental Health Team in the Schools* (1971), Lawrence describes the development and implementation of a mental health consultation program that was very strongly influenced by the psychodynamic point of view. Lawrence accepts Newman's (1967) belief that regardless of special professional training, all people doing consultation need to have a psychodynamic point of view in regard to the concept of human growth and interaction. In Lawrence's view goals of psychodynamic consultation are as follows: (1) to offer teachers help in becoming aware of children's hidden feelings, strengths, and needs as well as the nature of their development; (2) to assist teachers in the discovery of their own strengths, feelings, and attitudes and of the influence of these factors on the child's ability to learn; (3) to encourage, through teachers, greater creativity and productivity on the part of the children; (4) to increase consultants' knowledge of children in the school setting through their intimate exposure to the ideas and skills of educators. Lawrence tells us that the major talent of psychodynamic consultation is the ability to appraise and understand what one observes. Understanding is abetted by a knowledge of psychodynamics as well as an understanding of constitutional and temperamental differences in children and their effects on emotional development.

According to Lawrence, psychodynamic consultation emphasizes the development of strengths. A major way of doing so is ''emotional reeducation,'' a process in which old hidden feelings and needs stemming from conflicts are brought to the surface, where they are more accessible. Then, within the nonauthoritarian and supportive consultive relationship, consultees are helped to appreciate their own strengths and are thus able to relive historic emotions that had impaired their psychic capacities. When these old events are reexperienced in contexts of psychological strength, they lose their deleterious potential and the consultees are strengthened by the cathartic effect afforded by the issuance of the negative emotion and by the confidence gained in the knowledge that they have mastered another psychological hurdle.

As teachers grow in self-awareness, they are more likely to be sensitive to and responsive to the needs, problems, and strengths of their children. In view of Lawrence's strong psychodynamic orientation, it is not surprising that she stresses the need for consultants to be highly aware of their own psychology, which includes a knowledge of deeper feelings, motivations, and countertransferences.

Lawrence emphasizes that while her approach to consultation has many factors in common with psychoanalytically oriented psychotherapy, its intent is definitely not to provide psychotherapy for teachers; rather, consultation emphasizes the ego strengths of the teachers and uses their motivation to help them deal with the child's ego strengths.

Lawrence fully accepts Caplan's (1970) position that consultees need not be aware of links between their personal emotional problems and the difficulties of, in this case, the students; this allows for unconscious defensive displacement within the consultee, such that the consultant can focus on the client in the discussion while in actuality dealing with the theme interference that is upsetting to the consultee.

Lawrence strongly emphasizes the "female quality to consultation." Describing consultation as female, not feminine, she emphasizes that while it is aggressive it does not attack. It waits, abides, and is receptive to aggressiveness, complaints, fears, etc. Evidence of a particular child's strengths are brought to the surface and kept in sight, as are the strengths of the consultee. Lawrence goes so far as to liken consultation to a womb, accepting, stretching to accommodate, and supporting early growth, yet, true to consulting philosophy, the two blood streams do not mix and the potential for growth lies in the consultee.

A case description presented by Cass (in press) will illustrate one salient aspect to, and contribution of, consulting from a dynamic stance. The incident took place in an elementary school. The consultant had spent approximately 5 months meeting weekly with a group of teachers. It had become clear to almost everyone in the group that one particular teacher disliked a particular aggressive child more than his behavior warranted. Furthermore, the teacher's handling of the situation had resulted in the two of them getting into a pitched battle with no truce in sight. At one point the consultant was able to facilitate the action of the teacher's unconscious, and she suddenly blurted out that the boy looked just like her younger brother! At this point the teacher stopped her angry tirade, and she looked rather embarrassed and uncomfortable in the dead silence that ensued. Shortly thereafter humor saved the day in protecting her embarrassed ego, and it was possible to discuss at length the way in which her own countertransference was getting in the way of handling the youngster objectively and effectively.

Consulting from an Adlerian Point of View

Of those of the original psychoanalytic group, Adler showed the most interest in working with children of school age. Major contemporary advocates of an Adlerian point of view in school systems are Dreikurs (1968), Dreikurs and Grey (1968), and Dinkmeyer and Dinkmeyer (1976). The Dinkmeyers have outlined the way in which Adlerian psychology can contribute to school consulting. They outline eight propositions regarding Adlerian consulting; all advocate the principle that behavior is purposive and proper consulting will enable the teacher to gain a greater understanding of the purpose of behavior. Their propositions are as follows:

1. Behavior is goal directed and purposive. The Dinkmeyers illustrate this point by referring to Dreikurs, who has taught that the four goals of misbehavior are attention-getting, struggle for power, the desire to retaliate, and the display of disability. The authors point out that here the Adlerian approach is very similar to the behavioral approach.

2. Motivation can be understood in terms of striving for significance. There is less concern with what the youngster is doing at the moment and more with the direction in which he is moving. For example, misbehavior may result in punishment that will also result in greater prestige in the eyes of peers.

3. All behavior has social meaning. For this reason, the Adlerian consultant will attempt to gain as much information as possible on the social consequences of the behavior in question. Adlerians emphasized that social striving is not secondary but primary.

4. The individual is understood in terms of his phenomenologic field. Understanding that teachers have their own phenomenologic fields is as important as understanding that the child has one as well.

5. The individual has the capacity to assign personal meanings to experiences, to decide. Hence a youngster's behavior may appear to be inconsistent, since the youngster may act differently in similar situations, yet the meaning of the same situation may vary from time to time for the youngster.

6. Failure to function relates to the psychodynamics of discouragement. Discouraged persons do not see alternatives, and corrective interventions are best directed toward altering the youngster's anticipations. Youngsters respond to expectations; if they are negative, the youngster is likely to live up to them.

7. Belonging is a basic need. Adlerians point out that it is a mistake to forget that the classroom is a social unit and that youngsters within this social unit will respond strongly to social pressures. It makes more sense to try to work with these social pressures rather than try to deny or repress them.

8. Adlerians are less concerned with what people have than with what they decide to do with what they possess. That is, individual differences are strongly emphasized; notes on which approaches work best with each youngster ought to be a part of the youngster's permanent record.

An example of consulting from an Adlerian perspective is presented by Dinkmeyer and Dinkmeyer.*

*From Dinkmeyer, D., & Dinkmeyer, D., Jr. Contributions of Adlerian psychology to school consulting. *Psychology in the Schools,* 1976, *13,* 32-38. Used by permission.

Action	**Analysis**

Mrs. Smith contacted the consultant regarding Jane, a second-grade student. The complaint centered around the child's causing a disturbance in the classroom and failing to work up to ability. The consultant, after listening to the general complaint, asks the teacher to describe the situation which she finds most difficult.

Attack a specific problem, not generalities.

Mrs. Smith: Well, if she is given an assignment, rather than doing it she first visits with 5 or 6 children in the room.

Consultant: What do you usually do about this?

Mrs. Smith: I usually say, "Jane, get busy and take your seat."

Consultant: What does Jane do?

Seek to clarify. Focus on the psychological movement and the transaction between teacher and child.

Mrs. Smith: In a few minutes she's back in the same pattern. She never seems to be bothered and readily recognizes she shouldn't do this.

Consultant: It seems teacher and Jane have an agreement about their roles—Jane misbehaves and you remind her. Is it possible she does this to get your attention?

Seek to identify the child's purpose.

Mrs. Smith: That's probably true!

Consultant: Do you have any idea of what might be done differently when she gets out of her seat and starts wandering around the room?

Consultant seeks teacher's perceptions and her collaboration.

Mrs. Smith: I've thought about ignoring her, but I feel this is not fair to the other children to ignore her when she is disturbing them; and if they enjoy her company everything gets out of hand.

Teacher poses first potential solution.

Consultant: You feel ignoring wouldn't change the situation in this case?

Mrs. Smith: No, Jane enjoys people too much. (At this point the teacher was encouraged to explore other remedies. After some exploration, the consultant tentatively poses a new procedure.)

Consultant: I wonder how you would feel about giving Jane a choice about whether she'd rather sit in her seat when there's work to be done, or if she'd rather stand up.

Mrs. Smith: That might work. I've never thought of that!

Consultant: My idea is that frequently with children like Jane we are forced to react to her. I'm
wondering if, instead, we could get her to cope with
you by giving her a choice. The next time in a private
conference you could pose to her the alternatives of
working at her seat or standing for the morning. This
must not be relayed as a punishment, but as a choice.

*Utilize the therapeutic agent
of choice and the child's
capacity to decide to change
the consequences.*

(At this point the teacher and consultant explore other
examples of misbehavior. Emphasis is placed on observing closely times when Jane is functioning and
commenting positively. Consequences are to be balanced with encouragement.)

The Dinkmeyers summarize consulting from an Adlerian point of view
as follows:

1. A focus on dynamics and psychological movement rather than upon labels
   and static entities;
2. A concern for the pattern of behavior, the lifestyle, or characteristic
   pattern of responses;
3. A recognition that misbehavior and failure to function convey a nonverbal
   message;
4. Awareness that the consequences of the behavior point to the purpose;
5. Analysis of the relationship and interaction between teacher and child.

Consulting from a Behavioral Point of View

Behavioral approaches are practical, specific, and relatively easy to implement. Additionally, behaviorally oriented psychologists have tended to
deal directly with problem behaviors rather than dismissing them as "merely
symptomatic." For these reasons behavioral approaches have been particularly attractive to teachers, as witnessed by the very large literature (O'Leary
& O'Leary, 1972) of behavioral principles in school settings.

One example of a case will illustrate some features of a behavioral
approach in a school setting. This case, reported by Walker and Buckley
(1968), involved a fourth-grade boy named Philip. Philip's behavioral problems included verbally and physically provoking other children, not completing tasks, making loud noises and comments, coercing attention from the
teacher, talking out of turn, and distractability. Philip attended to assignments
about 42 percent of the time. He was in a regular class but was referred to a
class for behaviorally disordered children. It was noticed that Philip tended to
work well on programmed material but was rather inefficient when working
on more traditional seat-work assignments.

The first aspect of the program consisted of establishing a 40-minute treatment period, 5 days a week, that was divided into 10-minute blocks with short breaks between blocks. Philip was placed in an environment in which external distractions were kept to a minimum. Additionally, he was put on a point system in which he obtained points for discrete periods of time on tasks. These points could be traded in for prizes. Philip's attending behavior increased from 33 to 93 percent of each session, a dramatic although not an unusual increase for behavioral programs. After the boy's study habits had improved, he was transferred to a regular classroom and his teacher there was instructed in ways of continuing to reinforce his adaptive behavior in class. This transfer worked out well.

This case illustrates some of the elements of the behavioral approach. First, a precise baseline of the boy's behavior was taken, which provided a departure point for measuring behavioral change. Second, the stimulus environment was modified to facilitate attention. Third, the time units of study together with the reinforcements were precisely defined. Next, the psychologist and the teacher were very consistent in carrying out the program, consistency being one of the hallmarks of the behavioral approach. Here can be seen the positive orientation of behavioral psychologists: instead of directly discouraging disruptive behavior, they focused on its alternative, on-task behavior.

While behavior modification has found wide application in educational settings, a careful analysis of the literature on the subject shows that much of what has been called consultation is not actually consultive. Rather, in a large proportion of the literature a supervisory relationship exists between the psychologist and the educator. Most frequently the psychologist instructs the teachers and has the authority to evaluate their actions. This arrangement is understandable, since a primary aim of behavioral psychologists in schools is to promote skill development in teachers. Skills are best learned by the method of guided practice, a method that of necessity requires a teaching relationship in which the instructor has the responsibility and authority to consequate the trainee, yet the fact that the process is called consultive often leads to confusion and disappointment on the part of young behavioral psychologists who hope to emulate the success reported in these published articles within a truly consultive relationship.

Behaviorally oriented consultants must rely almost exclusively on their own stimlulus values as persons and on antecedent-controlled procedures. Effective behavioral consulting is an art not extensively written about. Knowledge of behavioral consulting styles comes mainly from one's own experience and from personal contact with individuals adept at this particular form of clinical enterprise. There is still much to be learned about the process and art of behavioral consulting, but some principles (Dorr, 1977) that seem to hold will be summarized.

First is the matter of language. Most behaviorists use behavioral terminology, which has the advantage of accuracy and precision. This is a major
problem when the consultant enters the school system, however, since many
teachers find behavioral terminology to be especially distasteful (Friendly &
Dorr, Note 1). Most successful behavioral consultants find that it is preferable
to use plain English whenever possible. Additionally, the use of mottos such
as ''catch the child at being good'' and ''accentuate the positive, eliminate the
negative'' has been found to be helpful in rapidly communicating important
behavioral principles. The abundance of animal studies in the behavioral
literature also raises another problem. Animal studies provide clear examples
of behavioral principles but are often offensive to teachers. It is best to avoid
animal references entirely.

Because behavioral consultants usually come from strong academic
backgrounds, they are usually adept at intellectual fencing, which, as a good
consultant knows, is to be very much avoided. Related to this is the problem
of lecture. Since behavioral consultants are often academically oriented, they
feel very comfortable with lecture. Many packaged behavioral training programs on the market today use good behavioral teaching strategies that include lecture, visual aids, and so on. However, lecture is usually inappropriate in the consulting relationship because it deemphasizes the egalitarian
relationship between the consultant and the consultee. Behavioral
psychologists are comfortable with data and often support their arguments
with tables and charts, yet, as Lindsley has pointed out, teachers are not
necessarily comfortable with this type of material; many behavioral consultants have won the battle but lost the war because of use of this form of data. It
is much better to refer to behavioral change in a youngster that the teacher is
particularly concerned about. The teacher will usually be much more open to
the use of behavioral procedures when a change for the better is seen in a
youngster.

In the recognition that the literature on behavioral consulting is rather
sparse, I developed, with the help of my students Bill Behrendt, Lisa
Friendly, Debbie Joseph, and Betty Yoches, a behavioral consulting model
that was intended to avoid some of the above problems (Dorr, 1977). This
model, piloted in classes for mentally retarded children, emphasizes the use of
an in vivo modeling approach. Lectures are kept to a minimum, and most of
the consulting takes place in the classroom, in which behavioral technicians,
trained by the psychologist, work directly with children. This arrangement has
the dual advantage of providing the teacher both with an additional aide and
with an effective model of behavioral approaches. As the consulting relationship warms up, the aide may help the teacher improve skills in behavioral
approaches by the use of guided practice. Since the goal of behavioral consulting is to help the teacher develop skills, and since the best way to learn skills

is through modeling and guided practice, this approach would seem to be particularly promising. However, it demands that the consultant and technicians "get their hands dirty," interacting in close quarters with all sorts of students. This stance is relatively different from that of most consultants, who because they don't see patients or students are able to retain a dignity of distance.

While behavioral consulting seems to be a promising way to help teachers help children, I feel that caution is necessary. Behavioral principles, properly applied, are highly potent avenues to behavior change. Unfortunately, when misused they can be very destructive, which is not the case with most other therapeutic approaches. For example, skillful Rogerians can be very helpful if they are particularly astute in understanding the emotional messages being communicated, but usually no harm is done if the clinical point is missed; the worst outcome is usually neutral. However, behavioral approaches misused can be destructive, as the few sensational cases that have been reported illustrate (May, 1975). Because the consultant has no power or authority to evaluate or correct the consultee, the consultant is placed in a particularly serious bind. The consultee is free to misunderstand and misapply behavioral percepts that may, in turn, harm a youngster. Fortunately, the Association for Advancement of Behavior Therapy is acutely aware of this potential and has actively developed methods for monitoring the application of behavioral principles throughout the country. Review boards composed of experienced behavioral psychologists are available to examine behavioral programs for technical and procedural factors as well as for ethical and humane concerns. Behavioral consultants concerned with the use or misuse of a behavioral approach can consult the local AABT chapter for assistance and review of programs about which they have concerns.

Consulting for Primary Prevention

Some school consultants attempt to work toward primary prevention, which can be done by consultation with administrators and planners who develop programs. Another way to aim toward primary prevention is through programs that communicate principles of behavioral sciences to youngsters, particularly in the elementary grades. The idea of communicating mental health principles in the classroom is not actually new. Loftus (1940, 1943) developed a large activity program in New York City to teach mental health, and Bullis (1941) organized human relation classes in junior high schools. Taba (1949) developed materials and approaches to improve in a group communication, and Seeley (1954) trained and selected teachers and school administrators to enable them to guide discussions of human relations in the classroom.

One of the most notable early projects was developed by Biber and her colleagues (Biber, 1961; Biber, Gilkerson, & Winsor, 1959; Cartwright & Biber, 1965). They attempted to infuse mental health and mental health principles into the entire school process. The scope and elevation of the project was extremely large, which of course, did not make the project amenable to evaluation, yet there is little doubt that many youngsters were helped through the project.

Ojemann (1961) has been working with colleagues since the early 1940s on developing a program to teach children a causal orientation to the social environment. Ojemann explains this as an understanding and appreciation of a dynamic complex and interacting nature of the forces that operate in human behavior. It involves the development of a flexible approach to life and the capacity to empathize with others. The approach assumes that when persons have greater understanding of the causal nature of human interactions they will be better able to deal with problems in social situations. The goal of the project was to infuse these principles in all aspects of the school curriculum. Ojemann and colleagues developed programs for teaching teachers to communicate this causal way of thinking to their pupils.

To understand the importance of this, consider a group of youngsters who regularly wait for their school bus together. The senior member of the group is also considered to be the dominant member of the group, and all discussions generally tend to center around the topic that the senior member wishes to discuss each morning. A new and considerably younger member of the group wants to have stories heard by the other people, but the senior member of the group feels that this is usurping the place of dominance and tells the youngster to shut up, thereby precipitating an angry exchange in which the younger child is driven from the bus stop. The younger child interprets this as meaning that the older child is merely mean and a bad person, without realizing that he or she also played a part in precipitating the altercation by attempting, as the junior member of the group, to dominate the conversation. The more the younger child can be helped to understand why people act the way they do, the more likely that child will be able to deal effectively with such social interchanges.

Another example of the utilization of a causal approach is drawn from the work of Ashbrook (1971, 1975), who developed a procedure for communicating the principles of reality therapy (Glasser, 1965) to first-grade children. Ashbrook, a member of the clergy and a psychologist, worked in the classroom with the teachers in the early stages of the project. The second-grade classroom was having some difficulites because 7 of the 26 children exhibited behavior problems such as aggressiveness, hyperactivity, shyness, negative self-images, and underachievement. Class discussions were held from mid-January to the end of the school year. In the first part of this project, the psychologist was leader for about 60 percent of the time; the second-grade teacher led at other times. Children were given "thought topics," e.g., "Suppose you had no eyes; what would you do?" "Suppose you woke up tomorrow and all the boys were girls and all the girls were boys; what would you do?" "Suppose someone gave the class two airplane tickets to fly to Washington to see the President for a day; how would we decide who would go?" They also evaluated their lessons; e.g., "Why do we bother studying phonics?" "What good is arithmetic?" "Does it matter whether or not you know how to read?" "How would you teach next year's second-grade class to read?" These topics provided enormous opportunities for discussing causal relationships on a very personal level.

One discussion regarding textbooks will illustrate the way in which children were helped to understand causality. The project encouraged expression of feelings, and the children expressed negative feelings toward their reading texts. The leaders asked, "Where do books come from?" Many children thought that they came from God or from their parents, but aided with a little information, they soon began to understand that special people, such as curriculum teachers and other special teachers, chose their books. The next question was, "How can these teachers be informed as to your feelings about these books?" After a long discussion it was agreed that it would be desirable to talk to the principal, but it was then pointed out that if the children had nothing to offer as an alternative it was unlikely that the books would be changed. Hence many suggestions regarding improvement of books ensued, which, of course, led to a discussion of the meaning of "better"; that is, should books be entertaining or instructive, or both? At the end of a long series of such discussions, the children had a somewhat better idea of the "whys" associated with the development and selection of textbooks.

Another project in communicating mental health principles to youngsters was developed by Roen (1966, 1967). The purpose of this program was to prevent emotional disorder through (1) fortification of the ego, (2) providing greater comfort in school, and (3) recruitment and spread of effect of the intervention. Roen and his colleagues developed a behavioral sciences curriculum that included factual information in the areas of psychology, sociology, anthropology, psychiatry, development, etc. Furthermore, many questions were asked to facilitate thinking in children, such as "List all the ways you are different from a rock" and "List all the ways you are the same as other children." Toward the very end of the course children developed an autobiography to emphasize their uniqueness as individual persons and how they were different from other people. This program was taught at the fourth-grade level. Replications were evaluated (Spano, 1965) that found that exposure to the behavioral sciences class significantly changed in the positive direction causal thinking and democratic behavior. Also notable is the fact that Spano found a significant relationship between causal thinking and social adjustment.

Consulting for Secondary Prevention

While a vast majority of school consulting time is devoted to tertiary preventive efforts, in recent years there has been considerable interest in moving up the prevention ladder. A significant example of a secondary preventive program is illustrated by the Primary Mental Health Project (PMHP) based in Rochester, N.Y. public schools (Cowen, Dorr, Izzo, et al., 1971; Cowen, Trost, Lorion, et al., 1975). PMHP was developed more than 20 years ago as a result of frustration with a traditional post facto approach to mental health problems of school children. The founders of PMHP, Trost, Izzo, and Cowen, formulated a procedure for early identification of youngsters manifesting school maladaptation problems and subsequently launched preventive efforts that included consultation with the school personnel regarding troubled children. This project has grown from a pilot in one small elementary school to a large, mature program of national prominence.

A model that evolved from the philosophy underpinning this project consisted of the following major elements:

1. Early identification procedures for screening youngsters in the first grade to identify maladaptation problems.
2. Utilization of nonprofessional child aides to provide direct helping services to troubled youngsters under the supervision of the mental health team (psychologist and social worker) in the schools.
3. Enrichment of the program by providing consultation by the project senior staff and extramural consultants to the mental health team, to the teachers, and to the aides.

While over 100 publications describe program and research elements of the project, the best single review is *New Ways in School Mental Health* (Cowen et al., 1975).

A consulting episode that occurred on PMHP is described here to illustrate the preventive stance of the project and to illustrate the contribution of consultation. The case involved a youngster of about eight or nine years of age who had been considered a very sound, mature, and promising student. However, in recent months prior to the consultation episode she began to be moody, withdrawn, emotional, and somewhat difficult to manage. On one occasion she left the line that was going to the lunchroom and was later found sulking beneath the steps. On other occasions she was observed to burst out crying or become tearful for "no apparent reason." The teacher was concerned about the girl and referred her to the social worker on the mental health team. The social worker interviewed the child's mother and found that the parents were getting divorced and that the child's father would be moving far away. The youngster was upset by the divorce, particularly since she would now rarely see her father. A child aide was assigned to the youngster, primarily to offer a sympathetic ear and lend support. Such an action was clearly consistent with PMHP philosophy. The child was clearly not "mentally disturbed," but she was manifesting the early signs of a problem. Properly dealt with from a crisis theory point of view, we hoped to at least prevent significant trauma, and to at best help her deal with the loss and separation in such a way that she would be strengthened.

Senior PMHP staff rotated through the various schools in a consulting relationship, and I was the consultant who had the opportunity of dealing with the problem associated with this case. The child aide was concerned that she was not "reaching" the child, that the child was not opening up to her, and that she was making no significant progress in dealing with the child's problem. Present in the consulting session were the child's teacher, the social worker, the child aide, and myself. The child aide asked me directly what she should do to be more successful in helping this child. While I will often give a direct answer to such a query, in this case I did not. Rather, we used the question as an opportunity to discuss some aspects of crisis theory and to focus on what happens to an individual forced to deal with a loss. I elicited comments and associations from the teacher, social worker, and aide regarding dynamics associated with the case. Our discussion had progressed for about a half hour when the aide related the following story.

She had been attending weekly sessions at PMHP headquarters on how to lead groups of children. On one occasion she was detained by a severe snowstorm, and as a result was very late for her appointment with the youngster that we were discussing. The youngster had been waiting for her for at least a half hour and was furious. The usually quiet, sweet, and compliant youngster angrily castigated the aide for being late, for missing the appointment that was "their time." She was irrational and stubborn as she heaped abuse upon the aide. The aide was very flustered and hurt by what happened and attempted to defend herself by saying that the main reason she was late was that she was taking extra training that would enable her to help the girl more, that she really did care for her, that she had no control over the snowstorm that made her late, etc.

In discussing this episode in the consulting session, it was clear that the aide was hurt and puzzled by what happened, which provided us with an opportunity for discussing the aide's need to provide direct help that could be objectively observed. It was very likely that the youngster was responding to the aide's lateness in terms of the dynamics of the separation. She had experienced the feeling that she could not trust her mother and father to be present when she really needed them, and now this warm and caring human being, the aide, had also demonstrated unreliability. The child was likely displacing her hurt and anger regarding the divorce onto the aide. As such, this was a golden opportunity for dealing with the youngster's hurt, perhaps by using a reflective procedure, such as ''You're terribly hurt that I let you down,'' ''You feel I've let you down,'' ''It seems like you can't trust anybody,'' or even ''It's almost like when your father left.'' Any one of these reflections might have opened up a floodgate of feeling regarding the divorce, the very thing that the aide felt that she had not been able to do.

Clearly, the aide was attempting to ''force'' the relationship with the child. Because of her countertransference reaction when the child attacked her, her usual insight and sensitivity failed her and she missed the opportunity to help the child at that point. However, in the consulting session we were able to discuss this case and suggest ways to use this episode in future sessions with the girl.

Fostering System Linkages

Many psychologists engaging in school consultation are strongly influenced by the community psychology movement, which advocates primary prevention through system change. Unfortunately, few systems readily invite psychologists in to effect change. Indeed, systems generally attempt to maintain the status quo. Hence in most cases system change is undertaken only as a final result of the relationship with the school system. However, Caplan (1970) has advocated that consultation programs progress whenever possible from client-centered case consultation to consultee-centered consultation and subsequently to organization-centered consultation. An excellent example of the way in which this progression in consultation focus can take place is illustrated in an article by Emiley, Grundle, and Zolik (1975). The authors describe a consultation program for a Roman Catholic parochial school system serving a community of approximately 150,000 persons. The school system consisted of 11 primary schools serving 3300 children. Prior to the involvement of the consultants, this school system had very limited psychological and social services. According to the authors, the rationale of the consultation program was that the best way to effect long-term consultation benefits was to focus on establishing and strengthening linkages within the system and with other helping systems to work toward the goal of rapid and smooth interchange of resources. The authors define linkages as ''the development of liaisons and relationships either within an organization or between organizations which facilitate the provision of services to clients or which facilitate the organization of more integrative and comprehensive services.''

Initially the Roman Catholic charities sponsored two social workers who provided case-specific consultation to teachers and parents on emotional and behavioral problems in children. The social workers felt a need for some backup support and approached two of the authors of the article regarding differential diagnosis and recommendations of these cases. These two authors, who were associated with community mental health centers, agreed to provide direct case-specific consultation with school and agency personnel. Their roles evolved several times, however, their focus shifting to augmenting the skills of the social workers and formally training them in learning disability assessment and remediation, and even later to helping the workers in establishing an experimental resource classroom for the educably mentally handicapped and children with learning disabilities.

As the program progressed the social workers became more able to handle a larger number of referrals on their own. School personnel became more receptive to assistance from the outside. Progress was made in linking the family to the school system through joint school−family conferences. Parents were encouraged to become actively involved as team members in designing remediation and behavioral management procedures both for the home and for the school. Principals received positive feedback on the program from teachers and parents and became more open to the consultation program.

The strengthening of linkages is reflected in Figures 2-1 and 2-2, reproduced by kind permission of the publisher and authors, where it can be seen that many weak linkages became moderate linkages and moderate linkages became strong linkages. The schools began to be less isolated as the threat to their autonomy was compensated for by the quality of the services that were provided to the youngsters. Indirect linkages opened up more communication with public and Lutheran school systems. There was a considerably stronger relationship between Catholic charities and the community mental health center. There was better communication among various schools, between social worker and principal, etc.

The major result of this consultation program was that individuals and agencies were communicating much more readily and sharing resources to the benefit of the children in need. Because the lines of communication were opened, the role of the original consultants became less important, which is the entire purpose of this kind of consultation: to eventually make the role of the consultant more or less obsolete.

These linkages were strengthened through various means. The first was the provision of high-quality mental health services for children in need. Second, the consultants spent many hours in meetings attempting to foster communication between various agencies. Representatives from agencies were invited to other agencies' meetings, and task force committees and meetings were also established to foster communication. It is important to note

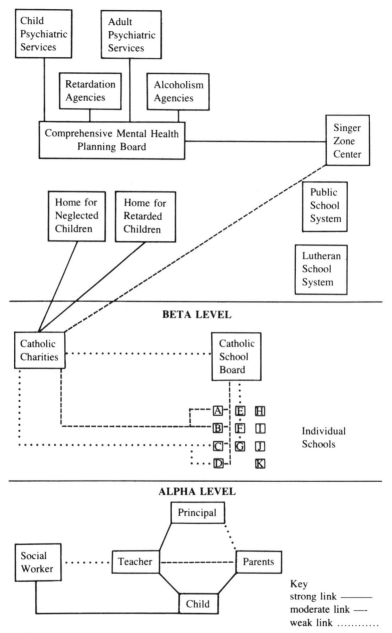

Figure 2-1. System linkages prior to consultation program. (Redrawn with permission from Emiley, S. F., Grundle, T. J., & Zolik, E. S. Community system linkages through a school consultation program. *Journal of Community Psychology*, 1975, *3*, 198.)

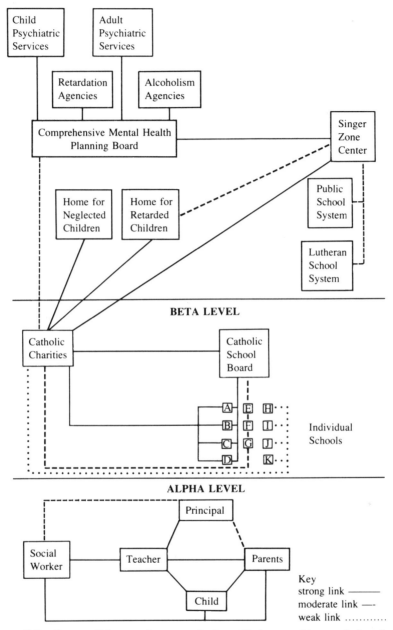

Figure 2-2. System linkages after consultation. (Redrawn with permission from Emiley, S. F., Grundle, T. J., & Zolik, E. S. Community system linkages through a school consultation program. *Journal of Community Psychology,* 1975, *3,* 199.)

that it was not necessary to form strong linkages in every single case; rather, some agencies and individuals preferred and/or were able to function with only moderate or even weak linkages. It is also important to note that this kind of system consultation did not take place in a brief period of time. A massive amount of time and work went into the establishment of this communication system, and progress was slow. There is no doubt, however, that the program resulted in more effective help for youngsters in the school system and to the system in general.

CONCLUSION

The waning influence of some major humanizing institutions, such as religious organizations and the family, have placed an even greater pressure on our schools to educate and socialize our nation's youth. This added responsibility is greatly magnified by the alarming increase in socioeducational problems such as the downward plunge in SAT scores, the epidemic of violence between teachers and pupils, and the dramatic increase in the juvenile crime rate. Many schools have been described as combat zones in which legitimate education is very difficult and the humanization process is almost impossible. Indeed, the chaotic conditions in many schools render their effect dehumanizing.

Society expects schools to be successful and is unforgiving of failure, yet schools merely reflect society, a society that seems to be moving in the direction of abdicating its responsibility to contribute to the humanization process. The entire burden is put on the shoulders of educators, and by many indices they are failing. If this trend is to be reversed, it is imperative that individual members of society, particularly those from the professional ranks, contribute their talents, skills, and industry to the educational enterprise, not in the form of meddling but in the form of support.

Psychologists are in a position to make enormous positive contributions to the process of education, particularly through the efficient vehicle of consultation. This process is very difficult, but if we can help children develop into brighter, better-adjusted, and more adaptive adults than we, the practice of consultation will be worth the effort.

REFERENCES

Ashbrook, J. B. *In human presence, hope; The pastor deals with individual and social change*. Valley Forge, Pa.: Judson Press, 1971.
Ashbrook, J. B. *Responding to human pain*. Valley Forge, Pa.: Judson Press, 1975.

Berlin, I. N. Some learning experiences as psychiatric consultants in the schools. *Mental Hygiene*, 1956, *40*, 215–236.

Biber, B. Integration of mental health principles in the school setting. In G. Caplan (Ed.), *Prevention of mental disorders in children: Initial explorations*. New York: Basic Books, 1961.

Biber, B., Gilkerson, E., & Winsor, C. *Basic approaches to mental health: Teacher education at Bank Street College*. New York: Bank Street College, Publication No. 62, 1959.

Bower, E. M. Education as a humanizing process and its relationship to other humanizing processes. In S. E. Golann & C. Eisdorfer (Eds.), *Handbook of Community Mental Health*. New York: Appleton-Century-Crofts, 1972.

Bullis, H. E. How the human relations class works. *Understanding the Child*, 1941, *10*, 5–10.

Caplan, G. *The theory and practice of mental health consultation*. New York: Basic Books, 1970.

Cartwright, R., & Biber, B. The teacher's role in a comprehensive program for mental health. Paper presented to the Fifth Institute on Preventive Psychiatry, University of Iowa, Iowa City, May 14, 1965.

Cass, L. K. Discipline from the psychoanalytic viewpoint. In D. Dorr, M. Zax, & J. Bonner III (Eds.), *Comparative approaches to discipline in children and youth*. New York: Springer, in press.

Cherniss, C. Preentry issues in consultation. *American Journal of Community Psychology*, 1976, *4*, 13–24.

Cowen, E. L., Dorr, D., Izzo, L. D., Madonia, A., & Trost, M. A. The primary mental health project: A new way of conceptualizing and delivering school mental health services. *Psychology in the Schools*, 1971, *8*, 216–225.

Cowen, E. L., Trost, M. A., Lorion, R. P., Dorr, D., Izzo, L. D., & Isaacson, R. *New ways in school mental health: Early detection and prevention of school maladaptation*. New York: Behavioral Publications, 1975.

Cowen, E. L., Zax, M., Izzo, L. D., & Trost, M. A. The prevention of emotional disorders in the school setting: A further investigation. *Journal of Consulting Psychology*, 1966, *30*, 381–387.

Dinkmeyer, D., & Dinkmeyer, D., Jr. Contributions of Adlerian psychology to school consulting. *Psychology in the Schools*, 1976, *13*, 32–38.

Dorr, D. An ounce of prevention. *Mental Hygiene*, 1972, *56*, 25–27.

Dorr, D. Some practical suggestions on behavioral consulting with teachers. *Professional Psychology*, 1977, *8*, 95–102.

Dreikurs, R. *Psychology in the classroom* (2nd ed.). New York: Harper, 1968.

Dreikurs, R., & Grey, L. *Logical consequences*. Des Moines, Iowa: Meredith Press, 1968.

Emiley, S. F., Grundle, T. J., & Zolik, E. S. Community system linkages through a school consultation program. *Journal of Community Psychology*, 1975, *3*, 196–202.

Glasser, W. *Reality therapy, a new approach to psychiatry*. New York: Harper & Row, 1965.

Glidewell, J. C., & Swallow, C. S. *The prevalence of maladjustment in elementary schools*. (Report prepared for the Joint Commission on Mental Illness and Health of Children.) Chicago: University of Chicago, 1969.

Gray, S. W. *The psychologist in the schools*. Chicago: Holt, Rinehart, & Winston, 1963.

Iscoe, I. Realities and trade-offs in a viable community psychology. *American Journal of Community Psychology*, 1977, *5*, 137–151.

Joint Commission on Mental Illness. *Action for mental health*. New York: Basic Books, 1961.

Kaufman, B. *Up the down staircase*. Englewood Cliffs, N.J.: Prentice-Hall, 1964.

Kellam, S. G., & Schiff, S. K. Adaption and mental illness in the first grade classrooms of an urban community. In *Psychiatric Research Report* (Vol. 21). Washington, D.C.: American Psychiatric Association, 1967.

Lawrence, M. M. *The mental health team in the schools*. New York: Behavioral Publications, 1971.

Lindsley, O. R. *Personal communication*. University of Rochester, 1972.

Loftus, J. J. New York City's large-scale experimentation with an activity program. *Progressive Education*, 1940, *17*, 116–124.

Loftus, J. J. The activity program in N. Y. C. schools. *Journal of Educational Sociology*, 1943, *17*, 65–124.

May, J. G., Jr. Moral, ethical, and legal considerations in behavior modification. In W. D. Gentry (Ed.), *Applied behavior modification*. Saint Louis: C. V. Mosby, 1975.

Newman, R. *Psychological consultation in the schools*. New York: Basic Books, 1967.

Ojemann, R. H. Investigations on the effects of teaching an understanding and appreciation of behavior dynamics. In G. Caplan (Ed.), *Prevention of mental disorders in children*. New York: Basic Books, 1961.

O'Leary, K. D., & O'Leary, S. G. (Eds.), *Classroom management: The successful use of behavior modification*. New York: Pergamon Press, 1972.

Parker, B. Some observations on psychiatric consultation with nursery school teachers. *Mental Hygiene*, 1962, *46*, 559–566.

Roberts, R. D. Perceptions of actual and desired role functions of school psychologists by psychologists and teachers. *Psychology in the Schools*, 1970, *7*, 175–178.

Roen, S. R. The study of behavior by children. In B. Gertz (Ed.), *Behavioral sciences in the elementary grades*. Cambridge, Mass.: Lesley College, Second Annual Graduate Symposium, 1966.

Roen, S. R. Primary prevention in the classroom through a teaching program in the behavioral sciences. In E. L. Cowen, E. A. Gardner, & M. Zax (Eds.), *Emergent approaches to mental health problems*. New York: Appleton-Century-Crofts, 1967.

Sarason, S. B. *The culture of the school and the problem of change*. Boston: Allyn & Bacon, 1971.

Seeley, J. R. The Forest Hill Village project. *Understanding the Child*, 1954, *23*, 104–110.

Spano, B. J. *Causal thinking, adjustment and social perception as a function of behavioral science concepts in elementary school children.* Unpublished doctoral dissertation, University of Florida, 1965.

Taba, H. *Reading ladders for human relations.* Washington, D. C.: American Council on Education, 1949.

Trickett, E. J., Kelly, J. G., & Todd, D. M. The social environment of the high school: Guidelines for individual change and organizational redevelopment. In S. E. Golann & C. Eisdorfer (Eds.), *Handbook of Community Mental Health.* New York: Appleton-Century-Crofts, 1972.

Walker, H. M., & Buckley, N. K. The use of positive reinforcement in conditioning attending behavior. *Journal of Applied Behavior Analysis,* 1968, *1,* 245−250.

Waller, W. *The sociology of teaching.* New York: John Wiley & Sons, 1967.

REFERENCE NOTE

1. Friendly, L. D., & Dorr, D. *An exploratory study of elementary school teachers' reactions to selected terminology from the behavioral, psychoanalytic, and humanistic traditions.* Paper presented at the annual meeting of the Southeastern Psychological Association, Atlanta, 1975.

Marshall Sashkin,
Theodore Kunin

3

Psychological Consultation in Industry

Psychological consultation in industry is a more complex topic than is readily apparent. This consulting is certainly not done only by industrial psychologists, but involves many whose original specialty areas were clinical, social, experimental, and educational psychology and, in fact, every recognized psychological specialization. Furthermore, most industrial consultants are not psychologists at all, yet their areas of expertise overlap with those of the consulting psychologist.

The problem of defining content for this chapter is that each consultant defines a personal field of competence. One psychologist may consult on wage and salary matters (as do industrial engineers and others), but another may have no involvement in this area. One psychologist might be involved in transactional analysis training (Jongeward, 1973) or even run transcendental meditation programs (Kory, 1976) while others would exclude these areas in defining the parameters of the field. Many consulting psychologists perform selection-related functions, but specific activities and approaches differ widely, and each individual's notion of consultation probably excludes some of what others do and includes something a bit different.

Another aspect of the problem is that there are literally no tools, techniques, or procedures that are legally restricted so that they can be used only by psychologists. More nonpsychologists than psychologists are involved with problems of selection, salary administration, training and development, statistical analysis, etc. While the label ''psychologist'' is, at this writing, protected throughout the country, the *content* of psychologists' work is not, in general, legally regulated.

We will exclude from our discussion psychologists employed full time by one organization, although many might be considered to be "internal consultants"; we will concentrate instead on the work of psychologists external to organizations. We will also exclude areas that are atypical, although the work of specific practitioners will sometimes extend beyond our arbitrary limits.

Definition

A dictionary defines consulting as "providing professional or expert advice." The field of psychological consulting in industry encompasses a wide range of advisory and service functions related to the behavior of individuals and groups in industrial organizations. It also includes a wide range of research work oriented toward resolution of industrial problems. The field incorporates the development and administration of surveys; the development and implementation of training and personnel development strategies; career development activities; executive counseling; and, most generally, the application of behavioral science to the resolution of business and industrial problems. Practitioners in this field help organizations ensure that human resources are adequate to achieve company goals and that these resources are properly developed and deployed, and appropriately utilized.

The Consulting Industrial Psychologist

What are consulting industrial psychologists like? The average* consultant is male (more than 90 percent), in his early 40s, and earned about $36,000 in 1975. He has a Ph.D. (about 15 percent have masters' degrees) and entered the field in the early 1960s. About one-third of all industrial organizational psychologists are full-time consultants; this figure has not changed much in the past 30 years (Canter, 1948; Tiffin, 1958). Beyond these bare statistics, there is surprisingly little that can be said about consulting industrial-organizational psychologists as a group. Based on the great diversity of activities discussed above, it would seem likely that many practitioners in the field are themselves "multisided," seeking work that is characterized by its variety. A diverse set of job activities is, perhaps, the clearest general observation that can be made about what a person entering the field might expect.

*Taken from surveys of members of the Division of Industrial and Organizational Psychology of the American Psychological Association, conducted by Ann Durand and Wayne Sorenson (1975).

Part-Time Academically Based Consultants

To our knowledge, no data exist giving relative proportions of full-time and part-time (academically based) consulting psychologists or giving comparisons between these groups. We can do little more than state some fairly obvious facts.

Our strong impression is that most academics do consult and most seem to do so on a rather small scale. They tend to be oriented toward short-range projects (e.g., management training courses and workshops), which is not surprising, and serve more to supplement the services of full-time consultants than to compete with them for clients. Academically based part-time consultants will be more likely to engage in projects with a strong research element, since the outcome may lead to publication (as well as income). Academic consultancy is a legitimate activity, and schools typically assume that faculty will take about one day a week for private consulting. Aside from income and potential research advantages, the faculty member gains by remaining in contact with up-to-date real-world problems and practices.

Need for Consulting Industrial-Organizational Psychologists

Do consultants really bring to an organization a set of useful specialized skills that are of benefit to the client firm? There is some evidence that in organizations using consulting psychologists there exists an awareness of specific needs that require specialized skills that the client does not possess (e.g., see Quitmeyer, 1961). Management recognition of the relevance of psychological consultants for assisting with such needs has come slowly, since the 1940s, but steadily. Wulfeck (1950), for example, noted that consulting psychologists were not used to any great extent by business firms, while toward the end of the 1950s, Tiffin (1958) commented on the large and increasing number of psychologists involved in industrial consulting.

There is no way to say whether or not the needs served by consulting industrial psychologists are ''real'' or ''valid.'' It does appear that needs for their services are *felt* by managers in organizations and that psychological consultants are seen to an increasing extent as appropriate sources of help.

Many companies do not utilize consultants of any kind. Some companies employ psychologists to work on a continuing basis. Still other companies cannot justify full-time psychologists on their staffs yet feel a need for expertise in these areas on a periodic or interim basis; these companies utilize consulting psychologists.

DEVELOPMENT OF THE FIELD

The first source of psychological consultation to industry was the physiological approach, a natural extension of the foundation of psychology (in nineteenth-century Germany) by persons who were primarily physiological researchers. Next came the psychological approach, which developed in conjunction with the "raw empiricism" of early testing and assessment. The third basic source to develop was the social-psychological approach, originating in the classic Hawthorne studies, growing in influence through its group dynamics focus, and currently powerful through emphasis on organizational change consulting.

Physiological Roots

Psychological history books usually start with discussions of Wundt, Helmholtz, Fechner, and other German academicians, who were concerned with studies of reaction time, the speed of nerve impulses, the functioning of the senses, etc. When Hugo Münsterburg, one of Wundt's students, wrote his seminal text, *Psychology and Industrial Efficiency,* in 1913, he appears to have been somewhat defensive about his perceived need for an applied field to counterbalance pure psychological research. Münsterburg is frequently referred to as the father of industrial psychology. His text dealt with adjustment to physical conditions, economy of movement, monotony, fatigue, learning, and buying and selling. Early consulting work in industry was centered on determining the effects on productivity of physical variables (light, heat, ventilation), the optimal spacing of rest pauses, the effects of noise on productivity, and similar physiologically derived topics. Münsterburg was still very much experimentally oriented; the difference was that he was also interested in the practical applications of what had been learned about human functioning (1917).

In somewhat more sophisticated form such studies are still carried out in a field commonly called "human engineering." This area, which has also been called applied experimental research, emerged from the Second World War, developing in the context of consultation to the military by Chapanis, Garner, & Morgan (1949) and others. The focus of human engineering studies is on the design of equipment to minimize operator error. The "man-machine system" is viewed as an operating unit, and studies are performed to maximize the system's effectiveness and dependability. On the mundane side, this work includes, for example, design of knobs and controls on washing machines. Occasionally, however, research is applied to solve more serious problems. A good example occurred a few years ago when it was noted that a larger than chance number of aircraft were crashing short of runways at night when all weather conditions were excellent. The researcher/consultants found the cause to be an optical illusion that occurs when a person is descending from a height at night. Normally harmless, this minor physiological quirk was costing lives when pilots were "fooled." Minor instrument modification and pilot training have largely eliminated this form of accident. Thus physiological studies are still with us, although they now constitute only one small aspect of the field of psychological consultation to industry.

Psychological Roots

During the First World War, psychologists contributed to the American war effort by applying their knowledge to meet the needs of the military establishment. Performance evaluation systems were developed. Training programs, based on learning principles discovered through psychological research, were utilized. In the Army, faced with the problem of making effective use of talents of large numbers of recruits, psychologists developed the Army Alpha, an intelligence test suitable for group administration, as a basis for determining the capacity of soldiers to learn and to aid in placement decisions. Since there were many recruits who were illiterate, the Army Beta, a nonverbal intelligence test, was developed. Personality inventories were developed as a time-saving measure in the psychiatric screening of recruits prior to induction. Trade tests were developed to evaluate the competence of recruits for specialized job assignments.

When the war ended, many of these techniques and procedures were carried over into industry. Aptitude and personality testing came into widespread use, albeit without proper controls, because of the need in industry for better selection procedures. Rating scales became commonplace in determining worker effectiveness.

This aspect of psychological work in industry continues to be a major work focus and probably is closest to the lay public's stereotype of "industrial psychology." Psychological testing has been refined and has edged toward becoming a true science. Even so, there remain problems of quality in application. It is not possible to say to what extent these problems are a result of improper testing applications by nonpsychologists. In any case, the recent concerns over discrimination through the use of psychological tests—a concern that has in some cases been proven accurate in court (*Griggs* v. *Duke Power Co.*, 1971; *Albemarle Paper Co.* v. *Moody*, 1975)—has made psychologists and managers aware of the requirements of valid testing and has probably reduced the frequency of improper applications.

Although tests and test validation procedures continue to be developed, researched, and refined, it was during the period between the two world wars that the primary emphasis of psychological consulting in industry was in this area, often called "personnel research." The aims included predicting performance, lowering turnover, highlighting employees with growth capacity, etc. At the same time, a new, third major area was in the germination stage. Oddly enough, this new work focus developed as a result of some traditional physiological research work.

Social Psychology in Industry

It was during the between-war period that a series of research studies was carried out under the leadership of Elton Mayo over a 12-year period starting in 1927 at the Hawthorne Works of the Western Electric Company. These studies served to change the future course of the field. Originally, the "Hawthorne Studies" involved a group of industrial engineers using the traditional physiological approach. Their aim was to determine the effects of environmental conditions on work productivity. While initial tests went much as expected, it soon became evident that something peculiar was occurring, since production increased not only as the level of illumination was raised in the test room but also as it was decreased. A group of "social scientists" took over the studies, the primary researchers being Fritz Roethlisberger, an external consultant, and William Dickson, an internal "personnel man." Their research demonstrated that productivity was greatly affected by factors other than physical working conditions (Roethlisberger & Dickson, 1939). Specifically, the informal social groups established by the workers—and the norms of behavior developed and supported by these groups—has as much or more effect on performance as working conditions.

The Hawthorne Studies first brought to light the importance of employee attitudes and motivation as well as the significant effects of informal groups. The final phase of these studies was focused on personnel counseling designed to help workers deal with their problems on an individual clinical basis and to help supervisors improve their supervisory methods (Zaleznik, Christensen, & Roethlisberger, 1958). The project was judged successful in improving personal adjustments, supervisor-employee relations, and employee-management relations, even though it was ultimately discontinued (Dickson & Roethlisberger, 1966). However, the primary significance of the Hawthorne Studies was enlargement of the field of industrial consulting by psychologists to include far more than psychological factors in work design and psychophysiological abilities. Psychological consulting to industry after the Hawthorne Studies encompassed the social behavior of individuals and groups.

The Hawthorne Studies raised management's level of awareness regarding the importance of social behavior in organizations. Later developments, arising out of group dynamics research, centered even more on the small group as both an operative team and as a training medium. The team approach can in part be attributed to increased technological—and organizational— complexity as well as to the spread of the view (among managers) that participation through groups is desirable. This view has been promulgated by many psychologists who consult in industry, perhaps most notably by Likert (1961). It derives to a large extent from the development of group training methods, in particular the "T-group" or sensitivity training group, an unstructured small group composed of about 8–12 people who typically meet for a total of about 30 hours with no agenda except to observe and learn from their own "here and now" behavior. The method was developed serendipitously by Kenneth Benne, Leland Bradford, Ronald Lippitt, and Kurt Lewin in a 1946 workshop. The first three founded the National Training Laboratories (NTL), which made sensitivity training available to industry. Many companies have utilized the NTL program and similar programs offered across the country. In recent years sensitivity training has fallen somewhat out of favor as a widely used consultation approach.

Surveys of social-psychological attitudes, inspired by the Hawthorne Studies, were very popular through the 1950s. The 1960s were the years of the T-group and of group training in a more general sense. From the late 1960s through the 1970s, still another thrust has developed, based on the two just noted, making use of surveys for gathering data and centered on the group as both target and agent of change. The ultimate aim, however, is *organizational* change, or, as it is commonly called, organization development (OD). Although OD has recently become so popular as to be judged but a fad by some, there are indications that it is in the process of becoming yet another stable focus of psychological consultation in industry.

CONSULTING ACTIVITIES

Based on the historical outline given above we can define three areas of consulting application and infer a fourth (Table 3-1). In each of these areas we can identify specific consulting activities.

The first area might be called "concern for individual-organizational fit." Included in this area are the activities of psychological assessment, counseling, career planning, and searching for managerial personnel. In addition, some individually focused training and development work would fit into this area of consulting application. Some of the activities mentioned need further definition. Psychological assessment includes the development and validation of tests, assessment interviewing, and assessment center activities. Each of these will be discussed.

A second area of consulting activity centers on groups or organizational

Table 3-1
Consulting Activities

Activities concerned primarily with individuals

Psychological assessment—evaluation of individuals through tests, interviews, and assessment centers

Career planning

Counseling—clinical, quasitherapeutic help in dealing with individual problems

Management search—seeking out and selecting middle- and higher-level managerial personnel

Activities concerned primarily with groups or units

Training and development—job training; supervisory training; management development; organization development

Surveying—development and use of attitude and organizational diagnostic survey instruments

Activities concerned primarily with the organization

Personnel systems development—construction, use, and validation of psychological tests; development of selection and placement policies and procedures

Reward systems development—design and implementation of policies and procedures regarding pay and rewards, including job analysis (determination of the comparative worth of jobs), performance appraisal, and specific techniques (such as management by objectives)

Activities concerned primarily with the relation between the organization and its environment

Industrial labor relations—dealing with union—management conflicts

Consumer behavior research—market research

---

units. This area, of course, developed from the early industrial social psychology approach. It includes much training and development work, particularly when such activities involve intact work teams. While organization development (OD) has an ultimate aim of changing the entire organization, it is in practice most commonly applied in medium- or small-sized fairly autonomous subunits (divisions, departments, executive teams, etc.). OD therefore fits best into our second area of consulting application. Another major activity in this area is surveying. Again, surveys may often apply to an entire organization but are more likely to focus on organizational groups and subunits.

The third category includes those consulting activities that affect the total organization, for example, the design and implementation of personnel systems, involving the development and definition of sound selection and placement policies and practices as well as short- and long-range manpower planning, or the development and operation of organizational reward systems.

Finally, we will take brief note of certain consulting activities that center on the organization and its environment. Specifically included are activities concerned with labor and union relations and consulting on problems in the field of consumer behavior (market research, sales training, etc.). While these activities are definitely not *typical* of psychological consulting, they are performed by psychologists frequently enough to deserve mention.

These four areas of consulting application are not totally separate from one another. The distinctions made by our four-way classification are given more for convenience of discussion than intended as a formal typology.

While the consulting activities defined and described here were included primarily on the basis of the authors' experiences and biases, there is some—very limited—literature about what psychological consultants to industry actually do. A survey of associate members of the Division of Industrial-Organizational Psychology of APA by Courtney (1975) provides some data. While these persons predominantly hold M.A. degrees, almost 25 percent of the respondents had doctorates. A comparison of those with and without doctorates showed few major differences in work activities. The largest differences were that those with doctorates spent far more time teaching and in attitude measurement and less time doing management development. (Almost half of the respondents were employed by business and industrial firms, while just under 17 percent were full-time consultants.) All of the activities shown in Table 3-1 showed up in Courtney's survey. Predominant activities were psychological assessment, surveying, training and development, and reward systems development. It is of interest that at least one of the activities in each category (except the fourth) was very common. Perhaps more interesting is the strong emphasis on individual assessment (including selection and placement at all levels) and on group-oriented activities. Courtney's (1975) comment about the great "diversity of activities engaged in by all respondents" confirms the image of the consultant presented here.

The Psychological Consultant As Change Agent

Before we proceed to define the activities listed in Table 3-1, we will briefly examine what we see as a general aspect of the consultant's role. In the broadest sense of the term, the consulting industrial psychologist is an *agent of change*. Being a change agent is part of the consultant's role process regardless of the content of the consultant's work. Whether the consultant is designing a comprehensive personnel selection system or conducting a few individual management assessments, one effect is the introduction of a change in the organization. This change may not even be intentional. The consultant represents an external input and has an impact not fully predictable by members of the organization. This typically gentle shaking up of the organization is, in itself, beneficial to the system, even if there is no obvious effect, and serves to get organization members thinking about the current state of the system in terms of desired (or undesired) changes.

Individual-Centered Consulting Activities

PSYCHOLOGICAL ASSESSMENT

Psychological assessment of job candidates or of employees considered for promotion or reassignment is one of the most frequent applications of psychology in business and industry. Typically, after a company recruits and prescreens candidates, an outside firm of consultants is used to provide management with an independent appraisal for more insight into the assets and liabilities of individual candidates. The consultant is expected to indicate the strengths and weaknesses of the candidates, to provide an estimate of their suitability for the job, and to provide some suggestions as to how the job should be structured so as to capitalize upon a given candidate's strengths and minimize the effects of weaknesses.

A typical assessment will be based on a combination of aptitude and personality testing, interviewing, and background and work history evaluation. Obviously, an effective assessment requires that the consultant be familiar with the demands of the job and have some understanding of the social "climate" in the organization. A consultant who has worked with a company for an extended period accumulates a great deal of information about how the client organization is structured and about the people with whom the candidate would be working.

While some very large companies employ psychologists on a full-time basis to provide assessment services, this is usually not economically feasible; psychological assessments are usually conducted by outside consultants. Some of those consulting firms employ university faculty members on a part-time basis to conduct assessments in locations away from the firm's "home base" when the number of assessees does not warrant a field trip.

There is considerable variation in psychological assessment practices. The techniques utilized vary as does the time required. Some consultants perform an assessment in half a day; others require several days. In some cases, one individual will be responsible for all phases of the assessment; in other firms, different consultants will become involved in various parts of the process. The relative weight put upon testing and interviewing will vary; some consultants use only one or the other. Some consultants routinely provide a feedback of the results of the assessment to the assessee, while others consider this a separate service that would be performed only at an additional charge.

Psychological assessment of the type described above should be recognized to be a somewhat controversial process. It is typically more of a clinical than a scientific procedure. What the client company has purchased is, in essence, a professional judgment; they may or may not be provided with specific test scores to substantiate the findings. While there have been numerous attempts to validate assessment procedures, results generally yield low positive correlation coefficients that are statistically significant when the sample is large enough. However, the typical assessment is not validated. While many candidates for many jobs may be assessed for a large number of companies by a given consultant, the number of candidates evaluated for any one job is quite limited and is typically insufficient for statistical validation purposes. Validation studies must therefore be carried out across job lines or even across company lines in order to provide a large enough sample for analysis. While there is much anecdotal support for psychological assessment procedures, practically no concrete evidence exists regarding validity or effects (Campbell, Dunette, Lawler & Weick, 1970). It is not unusual for a consultant-client relationship in this area to extend over many years.

A somewhat different form of assessment has gained much popularity in recent years—the "assessment center" approach (Bray & Grant, 1966). Most assessment centers involve a two-day series of test, interviews, and simulated management task activities (role plays, group discussions, "in-basket" exercises, etc.) during which each participant is carefully observed and rated by several trained judges. Assessment centers are usually designed for specific jobs. The participants are almost always current employees of the same organization being considered for promotion. It has been more than ten years since the assessment center approach was first used by AT&T. Since then the approach has been applied in a variety of organizations for numerous managerial jobs at various organizational levels (Byham, 1970; MacKinnon, 1975). Results are consistently positive in that persons assessed highly are in fact more likely to succeed in terms of salary and promotion than are those judged to have low overall potential, when the assessment center results are kept secret and not used for such decisions.* It seems safe to conclude that assessment center results can be valid predictors of managerial success when the center is properly designed and conducted.**

---

*A recent study by Hinrichs (1978) showed that informed judges using only personnel records made slightly *better* predictions than the assessment center.

**APA Division 14 has published a set of standards and ethical considerations for assessment center design and operation (Moses et al., 1976).

Concern with potential legal issues centering around the hiring and promotion of minority group members probably has had some stimulus effect on the rapid growth of the assessment center approach, but even the rarely validated traditional forms of psychological assessment have not generally run afoul of equal employment opportunity (EEO) legislation because they do not usually impact on a company's hiring practices with respect to women and minorities. The candidates assessed are typically being considered for exempt positions, and most candidates selected by companies to undergo the assessment process are white males. Furthermore, the selection decision, in every case, is made by the employer, not by the consultant.

CAREER PLANNING

Vocational counseling has been a mainstay of consulting psychologists for many years. In the directory of psychological consultants developed by the American Board for Psychological Services, Inc. in 1960, there are 66 firms listed that offered services to business and industry; 80 percent indicate that they do career planning or vocational counseling. Career planning is a new name for this field, and the emphasis has changed and broadened somewhat. Mid- and upper-level managers have become concerned about career paths and goals as a planned approach to personal development. Responses to this interest include a variety of self-help books and manuals (Dāuw, 1977; Ford & Lippitt, 1976) as well as increased attention to the problem from psychological researchers (e.g., Hall, 1976) and consultants. The concern of organizations for the career paths of members may be seen as an indication of an increased awareness of the need for greater "humanization" of work, or, more pragmatically, such concern may be a reflection of organizations' need to "track" and, if possible, control the level of commitment of members. That is, the more certainty the organization can develop as to the long-range plans of valued members, the greater the chances for effective operation in the long run.

Career planning activities are still on the increase in "popularity" at this writing. Based on Courtney's (1975) limited (and dated) survey, it would seem that psychological consultants were not involved in these activities to a very great degree. However, it is also true that most psychological consultants have had some involvement in career planning and are likely to become even more active in this area.

COUNSELING

Clinical psychological counseling has a long tradition in industry. One outcome of the Hawthorne Studies was the implementation of an individual counseling program, available to all employees (Dickson & Roethlisberger, 1966). There are, however, some basic problems with counseling programs.

If the program is run with full-time company-employed psychological counselors, these people have a conflict between professional ethics requiring absolute confidentiality and responsibility to their employer (e.g., when confronted with employees with problems that are likely to seriously affect their job performance). A logical solution might be to use external consultants, but this is not very common because of the high cost. A simpler and more common solution is to include mental health treatment in insurance plans.

Consulting psychologists do often act as clinical counselors at top executive levels; some even specialize in this form of industrial consulting (Argyris, 1976; Levinson, 1968). While such counseling may extend to nonwork life, it is probably more often limited to the work role. In sum, openly therapeutic and quasitherapeutic consulting activities are recognized and legitimate but also fairly uncommon aspects of industrial psychological consulting.

MANAGEMENT SEARCH

Searching out high-level management personnel is usually done by specialists in this field, commonly called ''headhunters.'' Some psychological consulting firms (e.g., Richardson, Bellows & Henry) have established search divisions. Usually, however, psychologists are called to consult on individual selection decisions. In that case, the consultation falls into the category of psychological assessment. Less often a psychological consultant (or consulting firm) will be asked to help in the search process. The consultant would then develop a set of viable candidates, presenting the client with options as well as recommendations. While this occurs frequently enough to be deserving of mention here, we emphasize that the vast majority of management search activities are carried out by personnel consultants who are not psychologists.

JOB DESIGN

Job design, redesign, or (as it was commonly called until very recently) ''job enrichment'' grew out of the pioneering work of Frederick Herzberg (Herzberg, Mausner, & Snyderman, 1959). Herzberg's theory of motivation was the basis for the practice of job enrichment—the redesign of jobs to incorporate more intrinsically motivating elements, such as sense of accomplishment, responsibility, etc. While the theory has been demolished by researchers, the practice of job enrichment has grown as empirical studies have confirmed its worth (Ford, 1969; Paul, Robertson & Herzberg, 1969). More recently, others have tried to identify the basic characteristics of well-structured jobs (Lawler & Hall, 1970) and to establish methods for rating jobs on these dimensions (Hackman & Oldham, 1975).

Job design involves the consultant in analyzing the content of a specific job with the assistance of managers and, in some cases, workers. Suggestions are gathered as to how the job could be changed to make it more interesting, to make the work activity a meaningful "whole" rather than a small piece of some larger activity, to add responsibility, and to increase recognition for work accomplishments. Worker participation is typically voluntary. The new job design, when approved by management and agreed to by workers, is instituted for a trial period. If results are good, the change is made permanent. This is, of course, a gross oversimplification of the process; a more meaningfully detailed description is given by Ford (1969).

Practically all of the work on job design has been done by academics who are part-time consultants or by internal staff members such as Ford (1969) at AT&T or Myers (1970) at Texas Instruments. Job design has become one major aspect of an increasing concern for the "quality of work life" (Work in America Institute, 1972).

TRAINING AND DEVELOPMENT

Training and development includes several different activities, some of which are centered on individuals, others on groups. It is important to realize that the vast majority of those involved in such training activities are full-time staff members, not consultants, and are not psychologists. There is a very large number of people doing this type of work; the American Society for Training and Development has over 10,000 members. Again, only a small proportion of these are psychologists.

Practically all of the lowest level of training—the training of workers in specific job skills—is done by internal trainers who are not psychologists. Psychological consultants, however, are often involved in the *design* of such training, which might mean description of a single on-the-job practice and coaching plan or could involve a complex situational simulation for skill learning ("vestibule" training) combined with content-centered presentations.

Psychologists are directly involved in training first-line managers and supervisory personnel more often than they are in training workers but, again, it is more common to find such training activities being conducted by nonpsychological in-house staff. It is at this level that "canned" or "packaged" programs are commonly found. These programs may require active involvement of a trainer in conducting demonstrations, using films or film strips, and even in giving prepared lectures. The trainer, however, is limited to the materials provided. This is intentional, since in-house trainers are typically not qualified psychologists. It is fairly common for psychologists to be involved in the production of training packages.

Some packages are intended for self-study and are "programmed" to a high degree. In this case programming refers specifically to the teaching technique made popular by B.F. Skinner (1968): after studying some materials, the individual is "tested," responding to a written question by choosing among several alternatives. Incorrect choices lead to remedial materials; correct choices allow the learner to progress to new materials. This approach is very useful when large numbers of people must be trained and when it is not feasible to train in groups owing, for example, to the need to keep many trainees on the job or, perhaps, to a great range in learning times among trainees such that an individually paced approach is required.

Programmed training packages, however, can be costly when job-specific content must be incorporated into the program; such a program might cost upwards of $100,000. Research shows that programmed learning is not, in general, better than traditional approaches when the quality of the latter type of training is in design and conduct equal to the former (Goldberg & Dawson, 1964; Nash, Muczyk, & Vettori, 1971). In some circumstances, the cost of designing a specialized program is then worthwhile, but this is not generally true. Programmed materials intended for general supervisory or managerial training, however, are relatively inexpensive when purchased from consulting organizations (rather than designed to order). It is fairly common for psychologists to be involved in the production of training packages of various types.

Management training and development, above the supervisor level, is more likely to involve the direct services of a psychological consultant. At this level it is not uncommon to find psychologists conducting as well as developing packaged programs. This type of training is most often intended to give managers a general introduction to behavioral science–based knowledge and to teach specific behavioral skills, such as effective listening or confronting and dealing with conflict. These programs are diverse in content and cannot be easily or simply described. Campbell et al. (1970), in reviewing management training research studies, used five categories:

1. General management or supervision programs—deal with broad basic introductory programs.
2. General human relations programs—concerned with interpersonal behavior, employee attitudes, communication.
3. Problem-solving/decision-making programs—deal with general skills and techniques for solving problems or making decisions.
4. Laboratory education programs—centered on development of awareness of one's own behavior and its effects on others through examination of one's actual behavior.
5. Specialized programs—oriented toward specific managerial job skills, e.g., appraising employees.

Methods are even more diverse and include lectures, seminars, sensitivity training, television, programmed materials, correspondence courses, movies, reading, cases, role playing, simulation games, and on-the-job coaching (Campbell et al., 1970).

There is ample evidence that management training can affect managerial behavior. However, the extreme variety of programs has made meaningful research very difficult. It is not yet possible to say that certain program content presented using such and such a technique is right (most effective) for a given situation. Even so, this state of affairs would be acceptable if we knew that professional psychological judgment made it likely that the right training approach would be developed or selected. However, the fact is that we do not know this to be true. Thus we can only state descriptively what exists in practice [and in very brief summary form; the reports of Campbell (1971) and Campbell et al. (1970) should be consulted for further detail].

Group-centered Consulting Activities

TRAINING AND DEVELOPMENT

As noted above, training and development may be group rather than individual centered. In this group context, the psychological consultant would generally be engaged in team building (Reilly & Jones, 1974), organization development (OD), or both. Team building is often one part of OD, especially when the team is the top executive group. Team building activities, however, may also occur at lower levels in the organization and involve intact work groups; such groups are usually composed of professionals (e.g., a team of engineers and scientists working on a research problem) or of managers.

Team building consultation is aimed at improving the ability of team members to work together effectively. While this may involve the team, as a unit, in some of the common management development training activities alluded to above, the most important aspect involves the consultant in helping team members to examine *how* they work together as they attempt to work on some real task assignment, which requires considerable skill in and understanding of small-group dynamics on the part of the consultant.

Organization development is a field of practice in itself (Huse, 1976). No brief definition can adequately express the content of an entire applied field. OD activities are tremendously diverse, but there are some basic elements to OD practice. First, the overall aim is to improve *organizational* functioning. Therefore while individual training may be a first step in OD, OD activities aim at more than just individual improvements. Second, and related to this first point, OD activities typically involve groups, usually groups of managers and often the top level of management as a group. Third, as is true of team building, the groups that are involved in OD work generally try to improve their own functioning in the context of real work activities.

As is true for management development, there are no clearcut research-based guidelines for OD practice, although some researcher-practitioners have begun to develop prescriptive frameworks (e.g., Bowers & Hausser, 1977). The research evidence on OD, while far from adequate, is clear enough to allow us to conclude that OD activities do frequently have positive impact on organizations (Friedlander & Brown, 1974; Frohman, Sashkin, & Kavanagh, 1976).

OD consulting probably involves as great a proportion of academically based "part-time" consultants as full-time consulting psychologists. One reason is that OD represents a "leading edge" of application since this field has only recently become popular (the term "organization development" was itself not invented until about 1960). The field has, however, become *so* popular that a large proportion of internal staff trainers and of external consultants have started calling themselves "OD practitioners," although their actual work may have little or nothing to do with OD. Two leading practitioners recently suggested that the term OD be abandoned, since "it has lost almost all of its specificity of meaning" (Jones & Pfeiffer, 1977).

SURVEYING

The work of industrial psychologists has long been stereotyped as the giving of tests (for selection and placement) and the construction and administration of surveys. In truth, the stereotypes are not without foundation; much of what consulting psychologists do in industry involves surveying.

Surveys may be simple or highly complex, and they serve a wide variety of purposes. Consultants of many disciplines use surveys to provide managements with information needed to understand and deal with the problems they face. Although psychologists may sometimes be involved in surveys of economic trends or of consumer behavior, we shall limit our discussion to organizational surveys. Such surveys are of two basic types—attitude surveys and organizational assessment surveys. The latter type has two subcategories—general data gathering for organization development and problem identification.

Attitude surveys of company employees have a long history, dating back to the 1930s. They constitute an efficient means of informing management about what employees are thinking. Surveys thus serve to remove some of the uncertainty around major management decisions that affect employees. Within the last decade, employee involvement and participation has become much more of a concern to management, perhaps owing to a more generally participative social climate. People seem less likely to accept without question what they are told by various authority figures. Surveys highlight current and potential problems, indicate their seriousness, and point toward areas where management action is required.

While the attitude survey can, of course, be conducted by company personnel, the use of an outside organization to guarantee anonymity and to provide an unbiased, "no-ax-to-grind" interpretation of the findings is a rather typical procedure. A knowledgeable consultant can help the company avoid many potential problems that could develop and can ensure that the company obtains maximum value from this technique. Many companies conduct these surveys on a regular schedule, utilizing previous survey results as a baseline against which to gauge progress.

There are consultants who spend the bulk of their time conducting attitude surveys. Others offer this service as a part of a broader range of consulting activities. The techniques utilized will vary from the use of "standard" surveys to the development of a custom survey for each specific application. In some cases, interviews rather than questionnaires will be utilized; in many cases, combinations of techniques are applied.

The practice of surveying has benefited from the fact that there are now a number of "standard" surveys available that minimize the cost of survey construction and that provide norms against which company results can be compared. Much of this development work was done by researchers at the University of Michigan's Survey Research Center, part of the UM Institute for Social Research.*

Science Research Associates (SRA), a subsidiary of IBM, publishes tests and designs attitude surveys. They have developed a "core survey" of 79 items that elicits employee attitudes toward basic areas of managerial interest and concern. The survey encompasses such areas as attitudes toward the company, toward supervision, toward co-workers, and toward working conditions, growth opportunities, rewards and benefits, etc. The core survey can be supplemented with standard surveys for specific groups such as supervisors or salesmen. Companies can also supplement with blocks of "custom items" designed specifically to relate to conditions or problems in the client company.

Typically, SRA provides the survey materials, carries out the data processing, and submits the printouts of the findings to the client. The SRA survey is probably the most widely used in American industry today, but there are other suppliers of these services as well.

The continued widespread use of attitude surveys appears very probable. Furthermore, managements have become increasingly sensitized to the negative consequences that can occur if the survey findings are not honestly "fed back" to the employees and positive actions taken. Effective consultants make sure that management is aware of the potential dangers and is committed to taking positive action in utilizing the findings.

---

*These researchers have produced two major "catalogs" of survey measures [Robinson, Athanasiou, & Head (1969) and Robinson & Shaver (1973)].

Attitude surveys attempt to discover how workers feel about the company and various aspects of their jobs. Changes based on the results would usually appear in the form of a company policy (e.g., supervisory practices, personnel practices, work rules, etc.). In contrast, *organizational assessment* surveys are aimed at generating data for use in problem solving and at pinpointing specific problems. Questions aim more at eliciting description of conditions than at workers' feelings. Analyses are commonly performed at the work group level for each group involved in the survey rather than summary data being reported for all respondents taken together.

There exists a very large number of organizational survey instruments; most consultants have their "own" survey. A trend over the past decade has been the development of standardized organizational assessment survey instruments, the best known of these being the Taylor and Bowers Survey of Organizations (SOO) (1972). The SOO is based on Likert's (1961) normative theory of organizations. A recently developed, broader survey instrument package is the Michigan Assessment of Organizations (MAO), created by Lawler and his associates at the Survey Research Center of the Institute for Social Research at the University of Michigan. The MAO has a core instrument and topical focal area instruments (e.g., job characteristics, conflict, reward systems, etc.). The core is used along with one or more of these topical questionnaires so that the MAO can be adapted to meet the needs of a very wide range of client organizations.

The MAO package is appropriate for consultation work around specific problem issues as well as for general organizational diagnosis. Questionnaire instruments like the SOO or MAO are very frequently used in organization development consulting. The data generated are typically shared with client system groups as part of the diagnostic process. Often, this takes place in a "waterfall" design, with each work group in the organization at every level, top to bottom, receiving and discussing its own survey feedback data. Very recently, Bowers & Hausser (1977) proposed that surveys could be used to diagnose organizational conditions appropriate for action-prescriptions *other* than feedback meetings (e.g., interpersonal process consultation, laboratory training, task process consultation, etc.). This use of organizational assessment surveys has yet to appear as a formalized practice, but the use of surveys to better identify and define problems within specific areas (e.g., conflict management or job design), followed by development of action plans other than survey feedback meetings for dealing with the diagnosed problem, is not new. In fact, the development and refinement of just such an approach is one aim of the MAO package.

Surveys can be useful and are used for specific (rather than general) problem definition, that is, without any organization-wide aspect. [Robinson, Athanasiou, & Head (1969) have produced a volume that catalogs, evaluates, and includes many such specific survey instruments.] It is probably even more common for individual consultants to create brief problem-specific survey instruments for a given client and situation. In summary, the skills of developing and selecting survey questionnaire instruments are of considerable importance for most psychological consultants in industry.

Organization-centered Consulting Activities

PERSONNEL SYSTEMS DEVELOPMENT

The basic task in this area of consulting is matching people with jobs. More specifically, in this category we include three major work foci. First, and most commonly known, is the consulting psychologist's development of personnel selection procedures through the selection or development, application, and validation of tests and interview techniques. Second, there is the broader and more basic work of designing and assisting in the implementation of personnel systems. Third, there is the organization-centered manpower planning study consultation.

Psychologists are often called upon to design and install selection systems that improve the selection "batting average" while adhering to governmental guidelines. They develop testing and selection procedures by reviewing current practice, selecting those parts of the current procedure that have merit and then building upon them. Typically, the consultant develops all necessary forms and materials required, trains company personnel in the administration of the program, and supervises its installation. The consultant with a continuing relationship with the client company can follow up to insure that the procedure is working as expected and to serve as a technical resource for the personnel department staff involved with the new system.

A great deal of consulting in this area involves validating testing batteries or selection interviewing procedures. The consultant may carry out the analysis of data provided by the client company or may merely design the validation procedures to be followed and interpret the results. The consultant may be called upon to testify that the program satisfies governmental requirements or to write to appropriate control agencies to offer a professional judgment with regard to the procedures used.

The development of a personnel system is a relatively "rare event" in the history of any organization and is usually the result of growth. When companies are small they cannot justify the expense of a personnel department. Personnel responsibilities are, in such cases, typically decentralized, and a number of key people are involved in handling various aspects of the personnel function. However, as a company grows, it reaches the point where a decentralized personnel function becomes cumbersome and decreasingly effective. Many psychological consultants are regarded as personnel experts and are hired to guide a company in establishing a centralized personnel function.

A typical procedure would be for the consultant to examine the company's personnel practices in detail, evaluate how well the various personnel activities are being handled, and identify those areas for which more sophisticated practices are required. The consultant might then be asked to develop improved procedures and to coordinate their installation. The consultant might be involved in establishing a personnel department, assisting in the recruiting, and, if necessary, the training of the personnel manager and in providing this person with support, if needed, until tne new personnel system has become established.

Typically, those areas examined would include recruitment and selection techniques, especially selection testing and interviewing, performance evaluation, reward systems, training procedures, promotion procedures, and employee benefit programs. The consultant might prepare a personnel procedures manual and serve as "midwife" to ensure that the interfaces between the personnel department and the rest of the company are developed in such a fashion as to minimize friction over the period during which personnel responsibilities are being reassigned.

The continued effectiveness and survival of any organization requires adequate human resources in terms of specialized knowledge and skills, but before it is possible to project future requirements the organization must have a "road map" for growth and development. The definition of such aims and the manpower resource needs that they imply is the purpose of an organizational manpower planning study. Such studies can be seen in terms of a stepwise process with at least four basic elements.

First, company objectives must be defined. The consultant interviews key managers to elicit their views of where the company is heading and what its needs are likely to be during a specified period. While five years is commonly used, the time perspective chosen will depend on the organization and its environment. For some organizations in environments of rapid change, five years would be an unrealistically long time span; for stable systems, ten years might be better. Management personnel throughout the organization, in addition to top management, would be involved in the initial data gathering process. The consultant pulls together all of this information, using his expertise to ensure that the goals and priorities arrived at are realistic. The culmination of this step involves obtaining top management agreement regarding the company's goals for the planning period.

The second step in the manpower planning study, defining needs, is started as part of the interviews and data gathering activities just described. The psychological consultant will, from the beginning, be concerned with defining the manpower resources needed by the organization in order to meet its objectives. When organizational goals have been defined, the consultant will aid in identifying the specific skills required by organization members, estimating the number of people needed, and identifying the key positions in various parts of the organization.

Once the goals and needs have been defined, the consultant will examine current personnel resources to determine the extent to which the organization may already have the necessary manpower resources. Personnel surveys, conducted at various levels within the organization, are carried out to estimate the growth potential of the company's talent pool. The procedures used to accomplish this will vary considerably from consultant to consultant, but some combination of a review of job performance measures, testing, background evaluations, interviews, and the elicitation of nominations from people at higher levels in the company will typically be utilized. At management levels, psychological assessments may be conducted. At lower levels, a "talent hunt" procedure will often be used. The result of this third phase of the manpower planning study is not only a delineation of the talent pool but also an identification of the gaps. Often a system is established to continue this procedure on an ongoing basis.

The fourth and final step in the manpower study is the development of personnel action procedures. At this point, top management has determined where the company is headed, what manpower resources are needed for success, and what resources the company has to work with. This next step, then, is determining, for each anticipated requirement, the procedures to be used to ensure that the needed resources will be available when they are required. In some cases, the company will be able to satisfy needs by developing present employees. In others, the company will have no recourse but to recruit new talent. In the former case, training and development programs will be established. In the latter case, recruitment schedules will be developed.

This information will be summarized in an action report couched in terms that have meaning to top managers. The process should involve the consultant beyond the report-writing stage, however, to ensure that the necessary decisions are reached and that an action plan is implemented. A report that sits on the President's book shelf has no value to anyone.

Not all organizational manpower planning studies incorporate all of the steps just described. The amount of work done by the consultant and by the client company's organizational staff depends on the situation and the company's internal resources. It should also be noted that all planning surveys are transitional. Once the reports are written, change will continue, and a year into the planning period the cumulative changes may warrant substantial changes in the plans. If it is well prepared, the program will contain within it procedures for continual review and updating.

The area of personnel systems development comes closest to the stereotypic public image of the industrial psychologist: testing for selection and placement. It is important to note that the consulting psychologist in industry is engaged primarily in the design of these activities rather than in giving tests and interviewing lower-level potential employees. The consultant examines, evaluates, and recommends new personnel practices; he determines the need for and design of a personnel function. He applies psychological knowledge to aid management in defining long range goals, determining future manpower needs, identifying potential talent in the organization for meeting those needs, and designing an action plan for obtaining and/or developing human resources for specific needs. The psychological consultant may, of course, assist in carrying out selection programs, in operating the personnel function, or in recruitment and training for resource development. These last activities are, however, more typical of full-time staff (some of whom may be psychologists).

REWARD SYSTEMS DEVELOPMENT

What is a job worth? Given that acceptable performance in a certain job is worth a specific amount of money, how can one determine the quality of performance of an individual and the consequent appropriate amount of pay? These are the two most basic issues in the development and administration of reward systems.

If an organization is to prosper it must adequately acquire, develop, and manage the human resources needed to carry out the many functions required for effective operation. Even if the firm is effective in locating and hiring the people it needs, in training them, and in utilizing their talents within a relatively efficient operating structure, it is still necessary that a system be established to determine appropriate pay for specific tasks and to insure that effective performance is rewarded.

Many consulting psychologists have therefore become involved in the design of pay systems and in the development of salary administration practices. While consultants in other fields, such as industrial engineering, also engage in these activities, a number of major psychological consulting organizations expend most of their efforts on salary-related projects. In fact, the most widely used system of executive job evaluation—the Hay system—was developed and is installed by a psychological consulting organization, Hay and Associates.

In recent years, the study of work motivation has received major attention from academic industrial-organizational psychologists (Lawler, 1973; Steers & Porter, 1975). This research has shown that people are motivated to work by a wide variety of rewards; some, such as feelings of completing a meaningful task, can be built into the job, while others are consequences of effective performance (as judged by superiors and by predetermined objective criteria). Rewards in the first category, intrinsic to the job, have only recently begun to be used in industry. The latter form of rewards is most commonly used by management, including increased pay, promotion, opportunities for training and development, recognition, special privileges, status symbols, and fringe benefits (such as deferred pay, stock options, extended vacations, company automobiles, etc.). While all are used to various degrees and in different firms, money is certainly the reward of predominant concern. Even when money itself is not a major motivator, it still serves as a "benchmark" for individual achievement. Dunnette (1965), a prominant industrial-organizational psychologist who is a consultant as well as an academic, has observed that organizations do not typically use pay as effectively as is possible to motivate performance. Nonetheless, organizations do typically *attempt* to pay employees in an equitable fashion, that is, in terms of their relative contributions to the enterprise.

Two basic factors determine what a job is worth. First is the complexity of the job and the demands it makes on an incumbent, as determined by a "job evaluation" procedure. Second, the scarcity or abundance of specific job skills affects the price that companies will pay for such skills. This supply and demand factor is typically measured by some form of *wage survey*. In addition, the tenure of incumbents is, to some extent, an influence on relative salary levels. In a union situation the extent to which seniority will affect pay levels is negotiated. In nonunion situations, the degree to which seniority will be recognized can be established by company policy which may be highly specific and tightly defined.

Many psychological consultants become involved in the development and installation of job evaluation systems. Job evaluation involves the establishment of common yardsticks along which diverse jobs can be compared. In effect, the variables used to determine pay are isolated, and rating scales are established by which the relative importance of each of these variables for each position can be determined.

There are many different systems for job evaluation, varying greatly in cost of installation and maintenance and in the accuracy of the judgments arrived at. The Point System and the Factor Comparison System (Otis & Leukart, 1948) are two basic methods of job evaluation with the capacity for a high degree of accuracy and concommitant high installation and maintenance costs. In both of these systems jobs are described, broken into components that are independently rated, and then "reassembled" to provide an estimate of total job difficulty. The Grade Comparison System and the Job Ranking System are methods by which jobs are evaluated as a whole rather than on the basis of their component parts. They are quicker and hence less expensive to use but lack the capacity for accuracy provided by the part-job methods. One of the consultant's responsibilities is typically to determine the specific method that best meets the needs of a given client.

The extent of active involvement of the consultant in a job evaluation program varies widely. In some cases, the consultant will carry out the entire procedure—create the necessary manuals and forms, study the jobs, prepare the job descriptions and specifications, rate the jobs, develop the wage curve, and design the salary administration program within which the job evaluation system will be utilized. Conversely, the consultant may merely advise management in the selection of the method to be used, train company personnel as job analysts, and coordinate the implementation of the job evaluation program. Either approach, if properly carried out, should serve to identify underpaid or overpaid positions, establish salary grades, establish a pay floor and ceiling for each position, and guide management in making salary adjustments. An accurate job evaluation system can help increase the motivational impact of pay.

When jobs have been evaluated in terms of complexity and difficulty, it is useful to obtain data about the value assigned to comparable jobs in other firms. Some consultants maintain intercompany wage surveys that they make available to the companies using their job evaluation systems. Although consultants are sometimes hired to perform a wage survey, literally thousands of wage surveys exist and are available for use as a frame of reference in setting the wage curve (Langer, 1975).

Performance evaluations (determining how well a given employee performs a job) are central to determining rewards as well as useful for other purposes. Training needs are defined, employees warranting consideration for promotion (or termination) are identified, and information needed for manpower planning is obtained. As a salary administration tool, performance evaluations indicate how quickly an individual should move through a salary grade and where, within a grade, a specific individual should fall.

There are many approaches to performance evaluation; once again, the time required and the cost involved are directly related to the level of accuracy that can be achieved with a given approach. For example, it is expensive to utilize a Forced Choice rating system or a system requiring supervised ratings. These methods both serve to minimize rating errors that can distort findings. Many of the performance rating systems used in industry today do not differentiate accurately between good and poor performers; such systems become a sort of obligatory ritual performed by supervisors, sometimes in "collusion" with subordinates. A poor system of performance evaluation can lead to demotivation of high performers and the reinforcement of poor performers.

Consulting psychologists are frequently involved in developing performance evaluation programs, in training raters, and in instructing managers in the application of evaluation procedures and policies. Sometimes consultants audit these programs, on an ongoing basis, in order to ensure that the ratings made are reasonably accurate and that rating errors have not become so prevalent that the system introduces more errors than it eliminates.

One particular type of performance evaluation program deserves special mention. Management by Objectives (MBO) is an approach by which performance is measured in terms of results achieved rather than effort expended (McGregor, 1957; Odiorne, 1965). Although the superior-subordinate goal-setting and goal-evaluation meetings forming the basis for MBO would appear to characterize the process as a more detailed performance evaluation technique, MBO can be an organization-wide system of management.

Top management develops organizational goals. Major department and division heads review these goals with their superiors and then develop objectives for their parts of the organization. This process is carried down to the point where all managers and supervisors participate in establishing their own objectives. Lower-level objectives must be congruent with those at the next higher level so that, if all goes as planned, organizational goals will be achieved.

MBO differs from other performance evaluation systems in that the objectives must be *quantified,* with acceptable performance levels established in advance. Furthermore, superiors share goal-setting authority with subordinates. At the end of the rating period superior and subordinate jointly review and evaluate performance results. One advantage of the MBO process is that it reduces the need for after-the-fact subjective judgments.

The system is frequently tied in with the awarding of bonuses in accordance with pre-established rules and practices. Thus an employee should be able to determine his bonus in advance based upon his achievements and company performance.

One of the advantages of MBO is that it forces people to plan their work and manage their time and effort in a way likely to produce the results that the organization is seeking. This system can have major motivational impact upon performance, but it can also have serious adverse effects if improperly utilized. As with other forms of appraisal, MBO can be subverted. For example, the goal-setting meeting may be a participative sham, with goals actually defined by the superior (Levinson, 1970), or people at various levels may lose interest and fill out the forms in a meaningless, mechanical fashion.

In the late 1960s MBO took on the characteristics of a managerial fad. MBO was eventually found not to be the panacea many consultants had claimed. Recent research, however, indicates that MBO programs can be effective and can retain their effectiveness if applied as an organizational program and if top management demonstrates continuing support for the MBO program (Ivancevich, 1972).

Organization/Environment-centered Consulting Activities

Three further types of consulting activities, while relatively rarely encountered (by psychological consultants), deserve brief mention—industrial labor relations, consumer behavior research, and quality of work life experiments.

The oldest of these areas is the psychological approach to industrial labor relations, pioneered by Stagner (1956), which involves a psychological approach to labor-management conflict. Stagner's work in this field started long before psychologists became interested in union-management relations and had a major impact on the definition and development of this field of study. Initially, this work consisted of research only, but there are now psychologists active in application attempts (Lewicki & Alderfer, 1973). Even so, this work today still has a predominant research focus, while persons active as arbitrators or negotiators, for management or for unions, tend *not* to be psychologists.

Consumer behavior research has been a growing field since the early 1960s, involving psychologists on a research basis but typically not in practical applications (such as market surveys to determine which characteristics of a planned new product should be "touted" most). While psychologists are employed by advertising agencies, the extent of their influence on marketing practices is quite uncertain [although folklore has it that much of modern marketing was an outgrowth of John B. Watson's (1913) behavioristic approach].

Finally, the most recent of these "minor" areas of psychological consulting centers on concern over the quality of work life (QWL), which some have termed "humanization of work" (Meltzer & Wickert, 1976). QWL consulting activities are varied, often involving redesign of jobs, restructuring of work using autonomous groups (work teams), and development of union-management councils to increase worker participation in decision making. All such changes have as their primary aims reducing the degree of alienation that workers may feel, increasing the degree and varieties of satisfaction workers obtain on the job, and benefitting the organization through improved management-employee relations and concomitant reductions in such cost factors as absenteeism, tardiness, turnover, grievances, and scrap loss. Psychological consultants involved in QWL programs are typically academics who "believe in" the importance of work life quality. In the U.S. (and Sweden, where a number of QWL programs are underway) managements—and unions—cooperatively involved in QWL programs tend to be those for which the latter set of problems is severe (for example, General Motors and the United Auto Workers), suggesting that the parties directly involved are acting less on altruistic or idealistic beliefs and more on pragmatic concerns (e.g., reducing absenteeism and retaining central control over "unruly" local union groups). QWL is at this writing, an expanding area of interest for industrial-organizational psychologists. If the area continues to develop, it is likely to attract more full-time psychological consultants.

Consulting Activities: Conclusion

If there are any clear conclusions to draw, they might be (1) that psychological consultants to industry wear many hats indeed and (2) that a relatively small proportion of their consulting activities have been statistically demonstrated to have benefit for client organizations. It is on this note that we turn briefly to further consideration of evaluation of services.

EVALUATION OF SERVICES

The differences in perspective of the two authors of this chapter are here highlighted. The university-affiliated author views each consultive activity from what is essentially a research perspective and evaluates each area of activity on the basis of its demonstrated validity. Certainly, the greatest part of the consulting of academicians involves the design of studies in accordance with "tight" research models incorporating hypotheses to be tested and statistical procedures by which the effects of manipulating the independent variables can be demonstrated.

The consultant in industry, however, functions in a quite different milieu, providing services by which a desired client objective can be accomplished. There are often no research designs and few control groups. If each project had to be carried out as a research experiment, the time and cost involved would often be prohibitive. The consultant devises an approach to achieving some tangible end, and success (or failure) is operationally determined.

The academician views anecdotal evidence with grave suspicion, while for the industrial consultant, this is frequently all the evidence there is. The academician tends to see long-term consultant-client relationships based on observed past performance—but with no research evidence—as a sham, perhaps feeling that the industrial consultants are charlatans and that their customers are certainly very gullible. The industrial consultant, however, would point with pride to many tangible accomplishments to which client companies would attest.

There is little clear *research* evidence that the various industrial psychological consulting services are effective. On the other hand, many companies are utilizing these services operationally in their selection, manpower planning, and personnel practices. The industrial consultant would feel that the lack of research evidence stems primarily from the fact that most of what consultants are doing is not research. Furthermore, the absence of research data is much more troubling to the academic psychologist than to the industrial consultant or to the majority of industrial clients who are buying services, not research.

There are reasons for the lack of research-based evaluation other than the desire to retain clients or the lack of research focus. One reason is cost, which can easily become burdensome for small or moderate-sized organizations. Another reason is practicality; in many cases research-based evaluation is simply unrealistic.

Let it be clear, however, that we are not stressing a need for research per se by consultants, however desirable this might seem in an ideal sense, but are rather emphasizing the importance of evaluation of services, and evaluation of psychological consultation services in industry is by no means ignored.

First, for many programs and procedures, especially those developed most recently, such as MBO and assessment centers, considerable research exists demonstrating effective applications. This allows one to conclude that the *procedure* does not require research or proof that it *can* work; rather, the question becomes one of ensuring that the program or procedure is implemented effectively.

Second, legal rulings requiring testing and selection programs and procedures to be validated for specific jobs seem to have had the overall effect of improving practices. Psychologists have taken strong initiatives in creating guidelines for the design and implementation of testing programs (Division of Industrial-Organizational Psychology, APA, 1975), and in the development of validated programs.

There is much room for realistic improvement in evaluation of service effectiveness. In achieving such improvements, it is neither realistic to expect psychological consultants to become researchers nor necessary for them to do so.

BECOMING A CONSULTANT

The single most important concern is selection of a graduate school. A good graduate school for the prospective consultant is one with a practical rather than theoretical orientation. The types and titles of courses offered are a good clue; a practical program includes, for example, courses on testing and on personnel techniques. A prospective student should also look for faculty who are active consultants, preferably having their own consulting firms.

Mayfield (1976; 1977) surveyed recent industrial-organizational psychology graduates and employers of recent graduates and found high agreement that the one thing students need most is direct experience with the practical aspects of business and industry. Faculty in schools with an active applied focus are aware of the need for real-world experience by students; in response they make efforts to place students in industrial internship positions and to involve students in consulting assignments or at least to take students with them on such assignments as observers.

Mayfield also found basic agreement by recent graduates and employers that more formal training in personnel selection and assessment and in performance evaluation and criteria development would have been helpful.

The nature and the breadth of psychological consulting to industry make important adequate psychological training in areas other than industrial. Much of the consultant's work has clinical aspects; a sound grasp of personality theory and variables (such as the nature and operation of defense mechanisms) is quite relevant. Understanding motivation—the needs—and attitudes—the frames of reference of managers and industrial workers—is also important. Even experimental design is of use in preparing project proposals.

The student can obtain more of a practical applied orientation by taking business school courses; many good business schools have industrial-organizational psychologists on the faculty (this is another place for the student to look for possible applied experience).

The authors cannot offer much in the way of detailed advice for obtaining employment as a consultant after graduation. The most common routes seem to be employment full time by an organization in the personnel function or full-time work with a large consulting firm. It seems fairly common for students to go to work full time after receiving a masters degree; many return for a doctorate after building a base of real-world experience that will serve them well when they are ready to become full time consultants.

CONCLUSION: ON BEING A CONSULTANT

The field of psychological consulting in industry is broad and fluid. The demand for such services has increased consistently over the past 50 years; the education of a manager at the undergraduate or graduate level is seen as incomplete without a basic exposure to industrial-organizational psychology.

Certain psychological characteristics and behavioral skills seem to us to be important for the consultant. First, there is the need to be comfortable working under pressure. Consultants do not spend a great deal of time sitting and thinking; they must generate client accounts, which means constant pressures for productivity. If one dislikes working under pressure but is otherwise very interested in consulting work, an academic position supplemented by part-time consultation may prove a satisfying combination.

The need to actually carry out one's plans, to finish in practice what one begins in concept, may also be significant. For the psychological consultant, it is not enough to analyze a problem and determine the optimal means for solving it; the solution must be carried into action.

Effective consultants must be able to sell themselves, which requires intrinsic self-confidence, since consultants often work in areas in which they have no background training. Effective communication skills are indispensible.

In time, the psychological consultant in industry acquires a frame of reference by working with a succession of clients. Psychologists working as consultants are not limited to practicing psychology; the demands made on them are broader than that. Most of their work is with nonpsychologists; they must learn to work effectively with clients by relating to their needs, adapting skills to the realities of a client's problem situation rather than trying to adapt client needs to their own discipline.

REFERENCES

Albemarle Paper Co. v. Moody, 422 V.S. 405, 1975.

Argyris, C. *Increasing leadership effectiveness*. New York: John Wiley & Sons, 1976.

Bowers, D. G., & Hausser, D. L. Work group types and intervention effects in organizational development. *Administration Sciences Quarterly,* 1977, *22,* 76−94.

Bray, D. W., & Grant, D. L. The assessment center in the measurement of potential for business management. *Psychological Monographs,* 1966, *80* (17, Whole No. 625).

Byham, W. C. Assessment centers for spotting future managers. *Harvard Business Review,* 1970, *48* (4), 150−160.

Campbell, J. P. Personnel training and development. *Annual Review of Psychology,* 1971, *22,* 565−602.

Campbell, J. P., Dunnette, M. D., Lawler, E. E., & Weick, K. E., Jr. *Managerial behavior, performance and effectiveness*. New York: McGraw-Hill, 1970.

Canter, R. R., Jr. Psychologists in industry. *Personnel Psychology,* 1948, *1,* 145−161.

Chapanis, A., Garner, W., & Morgan, C. T. *Applied experimental psychology*. New York: John Wiley & Sons, 1949.

Courtney, D. M. Work experiences of Division 14 associates. *The Industrial−Organizational Psychologist,* 1975, *12,* 33−35.

Dāuw, D. *Up your career*. Prospect Heights, Ill.: Waveland Press, 1977.

Dickson, W. J., & Roethlisberger, F. J. *Counseling in an organization*. Cambridge, Mass.: Harvard University Press, 1966.

Directory of American Psychological Services. Glendale, Ohio: American Board for Psychology Services, 1960.

Division of Industrial and Organizational Psychology, APA. *Principles for the validation and use of personnel selection procedures*. Dayton, Ohio: Division of Industrial and Organizational Psychology, APA, 1975.

Dunnette, M. D. A behavioral scientist looks at managerial compensation. In I. R. Andrews (Ed.), *Managerial compensation*. Ann Arbor, Mich.: Foundation for Research on Human Behavior, 1965. [Revised as: The motives of industrial managers. *Organizational Behavior and Human Performance*, 1967, *2*, 176–182.]

Durand, A., & Sorenson, W. Income of Division 14 members. *The Industrial–Organizational Psychologist*, 1976, *13*, 10–11; 1975, *12*, 26–28.

Ford, G. A., & Lippitt, G. L. *Planning your future*. La Jolla, Calif.: University Associates, 1976.

Ford, R. N. *Motivation through the work itself*. New York: American Management Association, 1969.

Friedlander, F., & Brown, L. D. Organization development. *Annual Review of Psychology*, 1974, *25*, 313–341.

Frohman, M. A., Sashkin, M., & Kavanagh, M. J. Action-research as applied to organization development. *Organization and Administrative Sciences*, 1976, *7*, 129–161.

Goldberg, M. H., & Dawson, R. I. Comparison of programed and conventional instruction methods. *Journal of Applied Psychology*, 1964, *48*, 110–114.

Griggs v. Duke Power Co., 401 V.S. 424, 1971.

Hackman, J. R., & Oldham, G. R. Development of the job diagnostic survey. *Journal of Applied Psychology*, 1975, *60*, 159–170.

Hall, D. T. *Careers in organizations*. Santa Monica, Calif.: Goodyear, 1976.

Herzberg, F., Mausner, B., & Snyderman, B. B. *The motivation to work*. New York: John Wiley & Sons, 1959.

Hinrichs, J. R. An eight-year follow-up of a management assessment center. *Journal of Applied Psychology*, 1978, *63*, 596–601.

Huse, E. F. *Organization development and change*. St. Paul: West, 1976.

Ivancevich, J. M. A longitudinal assessment of management by objectives. *Administrative Science Quarterly*, 1972, *17*, 126–138.

Jones, J. E., & Pfeiffer, J. W. On the obsolescence of the term organization development. *Group and Organization Studies*, 1977, *2*, 263–264.

Jongeward, D. *Everybody wins: Transactional analysis applied to organizations (rev. ed.)*. Reading, Mass.: Addison-Wesley, 1976.

Kory, D. *The transcendental meditation program for business people*. New York: AMACOM, 1976.

Langer, S. *Available pay survey reports: An annotated bibliography*. Park Forest, Ill.: Abbott, Langer & Associates, 1975.

Lawler, E. E. *Motivation in work organizations*. Monterey, Calif.: Brooks/Cole, 1973.

Lawler, E. E., & Hall, D. T. The relationship of job characteristics to job involvement, satisfaction and intrinsic motivation. *Journal of Applied Psychology*, 1970, *54*, 305–312.

Levinson, H. Management by whose objectives? *Harvard Business Review*, 1970, *48*, 125–134.

Levinson, H. *The exceptional executive*. Cambridge, Mass.: Harvard University Press, 1968.

Lewicki, R. J., & Alderfer, C. P. The tensions between research and intervention in intergroup conflict. *Journal of Applied Behavioral Science*, 1973, *9*, 424–449.

Likert, R. *New patterns of management*. New York: McGraw-Hill, 1961.

MacKinnon, D. W. An overview of assessment centers. Technical Report No. 1. Center for Creative Leadership, 1975.

Mayfield, E. C. Preparation for work in business and industry: Results of a survey of recent graduates. *The Industrial–Organizational Psychologist*, 1976, *13*, 30–32.

Mayfield, E. C. Preparation for work in industry: A survey of employers of recent I/O graduates. *The Industrial–Organizational Psychologist*, 1977, *14*, 29–31.

McGregor, D. M. An uneasy look at performance appraisal. *Harvard Business Review*, 1957, *35*, 89–94.

Meltzer, H., & Wickert, F. R. (Eds.). *Humanizing organizational behavior*. Springfield, Ill.: Charles C. Thomas, 1976.

Moses, J. L., et al. Standards and ethical considerations for assessment center operations. *The Industrial—Organizational Psychologist*. 1976, *13* (4), 41–45.

Moskowitz, M. J. Hugo Münsterberg: A study in the history of applied psychology. *American Psychologist*, 1977, *32*, 824-842.

Münsterberg, H. *Business psychology*. Chicago: LaSalle Extension University, 1917.

Myers, M. S. *Every employee a manager*. New York: McGraw-Hill, 1970.

Nash, A. N., Muczyk, J. P., & Vettori, F. L. The relative practical effectiveness of programed instruction. *Personnel Psychology*, 1971, *24*, 379–418.

Odiorne, G. *Management by objectives*. New York: Pittman, 1965.

Otis, J. L. & Leukart, R. H. *Job evaluation: A basis for sound wage administration*. Englewood Cliffs, N.J.: Prentice-Hall, 1948.

Paul, W. J., Jr., Robertson, K. B., & Herzberg, F. Job enrichment pays off. *Harvard Business Review*, 1969, *47*, 61–78.

Quitmeyer, C. Management looks at consultants. *Management Review*, 1961, *50*, 4–14.

Reilly, A. J., & Jones, J. E. Team-building. In J. W. Pfeiffer & J. E. Jones (Eds.). *The 1974 annual handbook for group facilitators*. La Jolla, Calif.: University Associates, 1974, p. 227.

Robinson, J. P., Athanasiou, R., & Head, K. B. *Measures of occupational attitudes and occupational characteristics*. Ann Arbor: Survey Research Center, Institute for Social Research, The University of Michigan, 1969.

Robinson, J. P., & Shaver, P. R. (rev. ed.). *Measures of social psychological attitudes*. Ann Arbor: Survey Research Center, Institute for Social Research, The University of Michigan, 1973.

Roethlisberger, F. J., & Dickson, W. J. *Management and the worker*. Cambridge, Mass.: Harvard University Press, 1939.

Skinner, B. F. *The technology of teaching.* New York: Appleton-Century-Crofts, 1968.

Stagner, R. *The psychology of industrial conflict.* New York: John Wiley & Sons, 1956.

Steers, R. M., & Porter, L. W. (Eds.). *Motivation and work behavior.* New York: McGraw-Hill, 1975.

Taylor, J. C., & Bowers, D. G. *Survey of organizations.* Ann Arbor: Institute for Social Research, The University of Michigan, 1972.

Tiffin, J. How psychologists serve industry. *Personnel Journal,* 1958, *36,* 372–376.

Watson, J. B. Psychology as the behaviorist views it. *Psychological Review,* 1913, *20,* 158–177.

Work in America Institute. *Work in America.* Cambridge, Mass.: MIT Press, 1972.

Wulfeck, W. H. The consulting psychologist in business and industry. In D. H. Fryer, & E. R. Henry (Eds.). *Handbook of applied psychology* (Vol. 2). New York: Rinehart, 1950, pp. 585–592.

Zaleznik, A., Christensen, C. R., & Roethlisberger, F. J. *The motivation, productivity and satisfaction of workers: A prediction study.* Boston: Harvard Business School, 1958.

Jonathan A. Morell

4

Issues in the Psychological Consultant's Interaction with Paraprofessionals

IN-SERVICE TRAINING FOR COUNSELING AND
THERAPEUTIC SKILL

The Need for Psychological Consultants:
Historical Context and the Present Setting

Many of the problems that a consultant may face in training paraprofessionals result from the unique factors that gave rise to the paraprofessional movement and that set the stage for particular frictions existing between paraprofessionals and professionals.

There are a very large number of social service and rehabilitation settings that employ paraprofessionals as counselors, therapists, and administrators—alcohol and drug abuse programs, halfway house settings of many varieties and purposes, community mental health centers, hotlines, and community outreach programs of all types, for example. The nearly ubiquitous use of paraprofessionals must be understood in terms of five factors.*

First, the use of paraprofessionals was spurred by the advent of several highly visible and influential self-help organizations. For our purposes, the most important consequence of these organizations was the popularization of the use of paraprofessionals and the establishment in the public's mind of the notion that treatment by paraprofessionals is viable and useful.

*This analysis is taken in part from an analysis of job mobility problems among paraprofessionals (Morell, 1975).

The second factor was a general feeling that self-help movements were far more successful than the more traditional professional treatment methods. Although this belief has been incorporated into the conventional wisdom, it is by no means necessarily correct; there is a dearth of methodologically defensible outcome research on these rehabilitation efforts.

The third factor is the generally acknowledged advantage of being able to relate to a client in terms of (sub)cultural background, personal experience, and communication patterns, i.e., to be able to empathize and to be able to form a relationship (Glasscote, Sussex, Jaffee, Ball, & Brill, 1972; Truax & Carkhuff, 1967).

The fourth factor to consider is the very fast expansion of rehabilitation services that has taken place in the last two decades, which has increased the need for social rehabilitation service staffing beyond the training capacity of traditional accrediting methods (Albee; 1968, Cowen & Zax, 1967; Peth, 1971).

The final factor, perhaps most important and least noble, is the cost of employing people with professional credentials. The social service system simply cannot afford to fill all possible counseling, therapeutic, and administrative positions with persons whose names end with Ph.D., M.D., M.S.W., or M.B.A.

Thus the current use of paraprofessionals stems from considerations of both treatment quality and economics. These considerations, however, do not operate with equal force in the professional and the paraprofessional communities. The firm belief that paraprofessionals hold in the usefulness and efficacy of their services is not completely shared by professionals (Andrade & Burstein, 1973; Cooper, 1972; Karlsruher, 1974). Much of the acceptance by the professional community of the legitimacy of paraprofessional service was undoubtedly motivated by economic necessity. The dichotomy is not complete, and there is considerable professional opinion in favor of the therapeutic usefulness of paraprofessionals. The debate does exist, however, and paraprofessionals are painfully aware of their less than total acceptance. [The problems and insecurities of paraprofessionals can be found documented by Levine (1975), Ottenberg (1974), and Rein (1975).] Anxiety among paraprofessionals is increased even further by their knowledge that social service funding priorities are in a constant state of flux and that the skills of nondegreed workers are not generally viewed as being generalizable across a variety of social service contexts (Morell, 1975).

Such are the forces that account for the present state of paraprofessionals in the social service system. Psychological consultants are needed to work with two related aspects of the training of these workers. First (and foremost) is the need to increase the quality of treatment that these workers give to their clients. Research from a variety of contexts clearly shows that empathy, understanding and a desire to help are not sufficient (although they may be necessary) to bring about constructive change in a client (Sparer, 1975; Truax & Mitchell, 1971). Second is the need to give paraprofessionals increased professional credibility and increased potential to apply their skills to a wide variety of problem areas. The consultant often must be able to accomplish these goals in a situation where there is an underlying tension between professionals and paraprofessionals concerning issues of status, salary, and power, conflicting opinions about who does the real work, and arguments about the skill levels of those who do that work.

It is, of course, not true that all mixed professional−paraprofessional treatment settings are battlegrounds. Constructive professional−paraprofessional cooperative ventures are quite common. It is important, however, to realize that the factors discussed here set up a dynamic that can easily lead to considerable tension between the parties. That dynamic is presented here in the hope that understanding might allow a consultant to eliminate problems before they start or at least to deal with them in a constructive manner when they do arise.

Conceptualizing Goals: Factors To Be Considered

The actual content of any training must, of course, be a decision reached mutually by consultant and employers. Depending on the situation and the inclinations of the parties involved, any counseling or therapeutic skill might be the content of a training program. There are, however, certain general issues that must be considered that cut across the boundaries of specific content areas.

Assessing the existing skill level of trainees. Consultants cannot assume any particular preexisting level of skill among their trainees—this is particularly important in the training of paraprofessionals, since strong feelings exist on the part of professionals and paraprofessionals concerning this issue. One of the motivating forces behind the rise of the paraprofessional movement was a strong belief by paraprofessionals that they held the key to rehabilitative success and that the techniques of professionals in the helping professions were of little use. The ideology stated that paraprofessionals had the necessary skills, that they were very good at exercising those skills, and that nothing else was necessary. Although this belief is somewhat dimmed today, it has by no means disappeared, and its legacy still exerts a considerable influence on the attitudes of paraprofessionals. However, many professionals believe that some or all parts of this ideology are incorrect. There are arguments to the effect that paraprofessionals do not have the skills necessary for the jobs they perform (Andrade & Burstein, 1973; Karlsruher, 1974; Sparer, 1975), and there is reason to believe that the skills that paraprofessionals do have can be improved considerably (Truax & Mitchell, 1971). Finally, one can make a strong case that the skills of paraprofessionals (such as they may be) are not sufficient to bring about substantive change in a client.* Consultants must have clear ideas of what they want to teach, of the extent to which the subject matter fits the existing skill levels of their students, and of the importance of the material to the work of their trainees.

It is all too easy to become swept up in the debate over paraprofessional skill levels and to find oneself taking an ideological stand. An unfortunate consequence of this process is that the consultant (i.e., teacher) may lose sight of the elementary fact that student abilities must always be determined empirically for each individual.

Who determines what gets taught? Trainees often have strong feelings about the usefulness of specific counseling or therapeutic techniques; this is particularly true in the common case of paraprofessionals who are themselves rehabilitants. Such people are acutely aware of the almost insurmountable difficulty of changing one's lifestyle, and it is quite reasonable for them to believe that what worked for them will work for everybody. These feelings are by no means unreasonable, nor are they necessarily incorrect. Furthermore, they may operate just as strongly for professionals who have spent many years learning and involving themselves in particular theories or approaches as they do for paraprofessionals who have spent many years in attempts to rehabilitate themselves. The problem for the consultant is that such feelings may make it very difficult for the paraprofessional to accept the validity and importance of a training program, and it may also be difficult for the consultant to accommodate to the perceived training needs of paraprofessionals.** Training cannot succeed unless there is clear agreement between trainer and trainee concerning the usefulness and the importance of the training program. To some extent such agreement must come about by negotiation and mutual agreement; however, a teacher cannot always ask students what they want to learn. There comes a point when the teacher, as expert, must convince the students that certain subject matter is important. The process of conceptualizing training goals must be a balance between mutual agreement and expert judgement. Such balance can be quite difficult to obtain with

---

*This is really an extension of the argument claim that any program designed to ameliorate social problems *cannot* do very much good (Rossi, 1972; Weiss, 1970).

**Although the author must admit that this dynamic can work both ways, he also admits that he strongly believes that the professional will usually be right. This attitude stems from his belief in the importance of theory, of systematic study, and of incorporating the implications of research results into one's therapeutic work.

paraprofessionals holding strong beliefs that they already know what is right. The best way for training consultants to handle this problem is to have clear ideas, before entering the training situation, of what is and is not negotiable. Consultants must also be ready to explain their positions and to have a well thought out rationale as to why they are right. (*Judicious* use of the power that comes from being an arm of an agency's administrative structure should, of course, not be overlooked.)

Specific skills or general theory.   A third issue in conceptualizing the goals of training revolves around the extent to which consultants should teach specific skills that can be put to use in situations arising during the paraprofessional's work life. Training programs can be geared to this level, and they can be quite helpful. An example of such a program is a "clinical case conference" in a drug abuse or similar rehabilitation program, where counselors present particular problems encountered in the course of their work. The goal of the professional-consultant is usually to help the paraprofessional deal with that particular problem. In a slightly less extreme (and far more common) situation the case conference consultation is used as a vehicle to give specific advice and also to supply knowledge that might be used in other, similar situations. The opposite extreme is to try to conduct a comprehensive program designed to teach general counseling or therapeutic skills, to explain the theory behind each technique, and to supply paraprofessionals with the knowledge to apply their skills to a variety of problems.

Several factors complicate the decision-making process on this matter. First, different techniques demand different amounts of theory as prerequisites to their successful application. Various techniques of client and case management can probably be taught in a relatively nontheoretical, context-specific manner. Behavior modification techniques are probably near the middle of the "technique—theory" continuum; although one could teach them divorced from theory, most experts would probably argue that some theoretical understanding is important and necessary. [For an example of a well thought out program that taught behavior modification to paraprofessionals see the reports by Suinn (1974a; 1974b).] Transactional analysis, Truax-Carkhuff counseling techniques, and various other group dynamics techniques probably also stand somewhere in the middle of the "technique—theory" continuum, and it would be advisable, but not absolutely necessary, to include some theoretical explanation in programs designed to teach these methods. One would probably find various psychodynamic and psychoanalytic methods at the "theoretical" end of the continuum. The important point to remember is that a consultant's decision on how situation specific to be is at least partially determined by the method of training chosen. As we shall see, numerous other factors must also be taken into consideration.

The needs of employers and trainees must also be balanced, and these groups may well have differing notions concerning the goals of a training program. In an extreme situation, an employer may want the staff to become generally proficient and highly skilled at counseling and therapeutic skills. Such a desire may arise from an interest in increasing the quality of service, improving the reputation of the organization, or any one of a number of other reasons. Employees, however, may be overworked, buried under an impossible case load, and not particularly interested in or able to devote time to a training program. Trainees in such a situation might be uninterested or might wish to use the program to learn some specific trick to make their work more efficient. People who need tools to solve immediate and pressing problems are not usually interested in how the tools were constructed or in how they can be applied to problems not specifically their own. Consider as a second extreme example a reversal of the interests of administrators and trainees. Employers may wish to institute a limited, inexpensive training program that would comply with an in-service training requirement that the agency must meet. Paraprofessional staff, however, may see the program as a chance to upgrade their skills, to gain some professional credibility, and to increase both job security and job mobility potential.

Obviously, the needs of all parties to a training program are usually not as divergent as these extreme examples. It should also be clear, however, that the needs of different parties for specifics, for generalities, for technique, and for theory can vary greatly. Part of the process of conceptualizing the goals of treatment must include a consideration of these varying needs.

Thus in conceptualizing the goals of training, a consultant must consider three issues with considerable care—the existing skill level of the trainees, the bias of the trainees regarding what techniques will be effective in their work, and the matter of how situation specific the training should be. Superimposed upon these considerations are time and manpower constraints, all of which must be combined to give consultants a realistic sense of what to expect from their efforts.

The Need for Training

Quality of service. The primary (or at least the most often mentioned need for training is to increase the quality of services rendered by paraprofessionals. Several important research findings become relevant to any consideration of increasing the quality of service by the training of paraprofessional clinicians. First, there is reason to believe that such efforts can be successful. Long years of professional training are not prerequisite to counseling or therapeutic ability. Furthermore, such work can be broken into relatively discrete sets of skills that can be taught successfully. (These findings have been replicated many times; see, for example, Carkhuff & Traux, 1965; Siegel, 1973; Suinn, 1974a; 1974b; Truax & Mitchell, 1971.) Second, although past personal experience with a rehabilitation problem may be helpful in work as a counselor or therapist, such experience is most definitely not sufficient for therapeutic or counseling success. Specific technical training is a necessity (Truax & Carkhuff, 1967). Third, experience and length of time as a therapist does make a substantial difference in one's ability to deliver effective therapeutic service (Karon, 1975). Finally, existing data present an unclear picture of the effectiveness of the clinical efforts of paraprofessionals (Karlsruher, 1974). In sum, it is reasonable to conclude that paraprofessional efforts at therapy probably do some good, that they do not have a marked impact on client lives, and that to some (probably small) extent the quality of service rendered by paraprofessionals can be improved through training.*

These data have important implications for the psychological consultant: they justify the need for the training of paraprofessionals by experts, they indicate that such training can indeed be useful, and they help one form a realistic sense of what can and cannot be accomplished. Training programs have been successful in increasing the quality of therapy delivered by paraprofessionals. In general, therapeutic efforts by paraprofessionals (and professionals too, for that matter) do not have profound effects on their client's lives. Thus a belief in the need for paraprofessional training must be based on a belief in the value of increasing the quality of treatment, irrespective of the "ultimate" effect of that treatment. Paraprofessional training programs must rest on a belief that the whole therapeutic-rehabilitation enterprise is in some sense worthwhile.

Professional credibility for paraprofessionals. Paraprofessionals, too, have needs for status, professional credibility, job security, and job mobility potential. All organizations have "organizational maintenance" functions as well as "stated goals" (Etzioni, 1969). Etzioni argues that these "maintenance" needs are legitimate and that it is a mistake for an evaluator to ignore them. One can make an analogous argument in terms of the "maintenance" needs of paraprofessionals and the paraprofessional movement. Paraprofessionals are in a particularly vulnerable and painful position in the mental health establishment; they are convinced that they provide useful service, yet they lack the professional credibility, training, and status that will allow them either horizontal or vertical job mobility. The problem is exacerbated by

*In all fairness, the effectiveness of the efforts of professionals in this area is equally uncertain (Meltzoff & Kornreich, 1970; Howard & Orlinsky, 1972), but the effect of therapy by professionals is not an issue in the present discussion. It is most likely, however, that as a result of training and experience professionals can render more effective therapeutic service than can paraprofessionals.

unstable social service funding and by the paraprofessionals' knowledge that they are the most vulnerable employees in times of tight money. Psychological consultants can and should try to meet the needs for institutionalized recognition of paraprofessional skills in the course of the training they provide. This can be done by two methods. First, college credit can often be arranged for successful completion of a training program. Many colleges (both two and four year) have a commitment to the cause of developing community resources and paraprofessional mobility. Furthermore, many programs train people at the bachelors and the associate bachelors level for positions in community psychology and the mental health delivery system. A suitable institution must be found and credit must be negotiated. The training program must be well laid out and relatively highly structured. Those who wish to receive the credit often have to pay tuition to the credit-granting institution. Participants in the program must be willing to work harder and more consistently than they would in an ordinary in-service type of training program. The consultant must be willing to at least equal the work and dedication of the trainees. These problems notwithstanding, it is often possible to set up such programs, and they can go a long way toward increasing the professional credibility of the paraprofessional mental health worker.

A second method of dealing with this problem calls for the granting of "continuing education units" as a method of granting recognition for learning outside the traditional "credit-degree" system based on the notion that learning is a lifelong, continual process that takes place in many contexts. One continuing education unit is defined as "ten contact hours of participation . . . in an organized continuing education experience . . . under responsible sponsorship . . . capable direction . . . and qualified instruction" (National Task Force on the Continuing Education Unit, 1974). To grant such units an organization (but not an individual consultant) must have a staff willing to administer and coordinate educational programs, bear responsibility for meeting the educational goals of the program, provide the necessary facilities, and maintain a permanent record of the continuing education units that it grants. Any structured learning experience can be granted an appropriate number of these units. Although continuing education units do not lead to college course credit or to a degree, they do represent an attempt at imposing a standard measure of recognition on learning that takes place outside of the traditional system of formal education. As a method of conferring professional credibillity, the "continuing education unit" is clearly second best to the system of granting course credit. Continuing education units do not lead to a degree, are not yet widely recognized as a measure of assessing a person's background, and are not yet coordinated by any single nationwide organization. The advantage, of course, is that the system is easily implemented, and it does attempt to impose some standardized measure on the educational value of in-service training.

Any employee, especially a paraprofessional, has a right to ask of an in-service training program, "What is in it for me over and above the value of the learning itself?" For paraprofessionals this right stems from their nondegreed status and from their extremely tenuous job security in the face of ever-changing priorities for social service funding.

Uses and Limits of In-Service Training

It is not likely that any of the parties to an in-service training program have carefully thought out the goals of the program prior to calling in a consultant to do the training. One of the consultant's duties must be to help articulate the uses to which the program will be put. The effects of poor goal definition are generally subtle and insidious. Most in-service training programs are not crucial to the actual functioning of an agency. How well counselors perform their tasks will probably have minimal impact on the existence and functioning of an established institution. It is not a trivial matter, however, if employees feel that their time is being wasted, if people dedicated to the cause of social service feel that the system is not responsible to the needs of the people, or if administrators feel that their organization is not operating at a desired level of efficiency. These factors make themselves felt in low morale, in friction between administrators and employees, and perhaps in lower quality of service to clients. In-service training programs can alleviate these types of problems by pursuing limited objectives in areas that relate either to the work of an agency or the needs of its staff.

As instructive examples one might consider some of the most common objectives of in-service training programs—an increase in the knowledge of an agency's staff concerning some specific topic, the teaching of some specific counseling or therapeutic method, greater employee job satisfaction, professional credibility for paraprofessionals, increased prestige for the agency that can boast of having in-service programs, and the meeting of the requirements of funding agencies. Clearly each of these objectives imposes a different set of requirements on the consultant and on the training delivered. Any number of these goals may be present to varying degrees in any training situation, and any given objective may not be shared by all parties involved. It must also be remembered that no matter what happens in the training program the agency will continue to function.

A consequence of having an inflated sense of the importance of one's work is an inability to set realistic goals. Unrealistic goals in the present context center on three elements: the effects of one's actions on an agency's continued existence, large increases on the ability of an agency to help its clients, and large increases in the ability and professional credibility of paraprofessionals. It is quite likely that administrators of employees in a social service agency may have these types of unobtainable objectives in mind when a consultant first arrives on the scene. It is also likely that there is little agreement among those involved concerning the importance of the various objectives that a training program might have. Thus the consultant's first task is to discover what is wanted by all parties, to assess whether or not those demands are realistic, and to impose a sense of the possible on all involved.

THE CONSULTANT AS RESEARCHER AND EVALUATOR

Consultants often find themselves in the position of having to evaluate or research some element of a social service system, which presents inherent difficulties and frictions that can be reduced only if the consultant understands the reasons for the problems. Many of these problems are exacerbated when an interface between professional consultants and paraprofessionals is involved.

The Structural Nature of Agency–Researcher Frictions

Friction between social service agencies and social scientists has been dealt with by many authors (Aranson & Sherwood, 1967; Bergen, 1969; Bloom, 1972; Caro, 1971; Fairweather, 1967; Fringe, 1952; Mann, 1965; Rodman & Kalodny, 1964). These diverse analyses have been organized into a systematic typology by Morell (1975).

Three elements account for the fact that social service agencies and social scientists often find themselves working closely together. The first of these factors is mutual need. Social scientists have developed a very large number of theories, ideas, and hypotheses that bear upon issues that concern social agencies; this research effort has developed a momentum that carries with it internal forces through which the effort perpetuates itself. Although there are competing theories of exactly what the "dynamic of self perpetuation" is, and how it works, there is general agreement that such a process does exist and that popular trends in scientific research do not die easily. [Two of the best starting places for a study in depth of these matters are Lakatos & Musgrave (1970) and Kuhn (1970).] For their part, social service agencies (presumably) attempt to maximize the benefits of their services, and in the long run such an optimization cannot take place without the help of social scientists. As examples one need only look at the contributions that research has made to the development of various counseling and therapy techniques and to the understanding of psychological phenomena that relate to the practice of clinical psychology. [See, for example, Rimm & Masters (1974) and Wolman 1965).]

More importantly (or at least more immediately), administrators are likely to perceive their agencies' funding to be related to the quality of service that their organization can demonstrate. Thus both social scientists and the personnel of social service agencies have reasons to work with each other, and hence the mutual need that serves to draw the parties into contact and cooperation.

The second force that draws social scientists and social agencies together is the force of tradition. We tend to believe that Science is a powerful and useful tool with the potential to solve many (if not all) of our problems. A consequence of this belief is that considerable prestige devolves to one who is associated with the use and furthering of the Scientific Endeavor. A second commonly held belief is the notion that one should try to help solve social problems if one can. [Psychology's commitment to this belief is well illustrated by Lipsey (1974).] These generally held norms are not lost to members of either the social service or the social science professions, hence a second pressure for social service—social science cooperation.

The third element that accounts for close researcher—agency contact and, perhaps, the most important is that belief in the usefulness of applying research to social problems is held not only by researchers, agency personnel, and the general public, but also by those who have financial control over both research and social service. These financial pressures impose a cooperation between agencies and researchers that touches far more topics than might suit either of the cooperating parties. Almost all evaluators have their private horror stories about having to research the unresearchable. Similarly, most administrators, counselors, and therapists have their complaints about being forced to cooperate in research that they considered trivial, uninteresting, or destructive.

In essence the forces of mutual need, tradition, and financial pressure have imposed between the parties a marriage of convenience that might not otherwise exist. It is but a marriage of convenience because the real needs and interests of social agencies and of researchers are quite different. The immediate needs of any social service agency are to maintain a smoothly running organization, to maintain fiscal integrity, to provide as much service as possible with limited financing, and to convince funding institutions that the agency is a viable and worthwhile organization. Such goals do not fit easily with research design that disrupts agency functioning, with concerns over long-range effectiveness, with feedback that is far from immediate, with allowing outsiders to view day-to-day problems, or with the scrutiny of rigorous evaluation; it is precisely these elements that are often embodied in the actions of social researchers.

Other problems also exist. Researchers tend to look for generality and similarity between discrete events or people (Bloom, 1972). Social service, on the other hand, is usually concerned with the immediate and specific needs of individual cases. Inherent in the notions of research is a force toward development and change; inherent in the administration of an agency are efforts at maintaining a steady state in the organization (Caro, 1971). A researcher's status is bound up with the process of discovery; a practitioner's status is bound to helping individuals by the application of a specific body of knowledge. Administrators (both professional and paraprofessional) gain status by maintaining a smoothly running organization; researchers gain status by publishing (Bergen, 1969). There are also different perspectives concerning the ethics and usefulness of control groups, randomization, and other accouterments of experimental design. Finally, there is a large difference concerning how researchers and social agency personnel conceptualize their work. The immediate interest of researchers is the causal relationship that exists between dependent and independent variables. One is tempted to believe that such information is also of considerable importance to administrators and to practitioners because such information can be easily translated into the issue of what effects an organization is having on meeting its stated goals. The catch in this argument is that attainment of "ultimate" program goals is probably not the real, practical, everyday concern of administrators or service delivery personnel. The daily concerns of such people probably revolves around surmounting the day-to-day problems and crises that always tend to arise. Thus the immediate concerns of social scientists tend to be the distant concerns of social service agency personnel, and nobody likes to be pushed into a confrontation with long-range goals when one is enmeshed in the daily battle for survival.

For all these reasons, social researchers and social service personnel form two separate communities with different norms, goals, and interests, yet they are pushed into a close association by mutual need, by the force of tradition, and by economic necessity.

Special Problems of Researcher—Paraprofessional Relations as a Function of Service Agency—Researcher Frictions

Special aspects of the paraprofessional's relationship with research consultants. The analysis presented above can be used to help understand the special frictions that exist between the psychological consultant as researcher-evaluator and the paraprofessional staff of social service agencies. The problems are qualitatively the same for all researcher—agency interactions, but they tend to increase in severity when paraprofessionals are involved. This occurrence can be explained by a consideration of three factors. First, although there are frictions between researchers and service agency personnel, there is a great deal of individual variation in any given person's attitudes about the value of research. Second, our school system presents a highly positive picture of the value and use of science. Thus positive attitudes about science are very likely (at least in part) a function of the length of time a person has been exposed to the formal educational system. Third, if a social service agency does employ paraprofessionals, it is quite likely that they will be found in counseling and direct service positions rather than in administrative positions.*

The role that factors unique to paraprofessionals play in the general analysis of research–agency problems. Researchers often view service agencies as the only laboratories in which certain important and interesting problems can be studied. It is quite likely that paraprofessionals will have even less sympathy for this view than other members of the social service community. This lack of sympathy is merely an outgrowth of the facts that paraprofessionals tend to have spent comparatively little time in the educational system and that the educational system is a strong force in shaping positive attitudes about science and research.

Although social science research has unquestionably made many contributions to the effectiveness of service agency operation, it is not likely that these contributions are recognized equally by all members of the social service community. The uses and advantages of research discoveries tend to be communicated in professional journals and conferences. Moreover, these methods of communication tend to be used by people who already believe that useful information is to be gained from scientific research. Social service professionals and research professionals may read different journals and attend different conferences, but some crossover is inevitable; in any case they share a general belief that information gained from research is worthy of attention. Professionals, by virtue of their schooling, are socialized into a system that continually reinforces them for dealing with innovation. Paraprofessionals are certainly not excluded from this belief system; however, they have had considerably less exposure to it.

Another factor that accounts for differing perspectives on research among service agency personnel is the role that an individual plays in the service organization. Although the funding of an agency is of vital concern to all its members, assuring continued funding is the responsibility of administrators, and administrators tend to be recruited from the ranks of professionals. We have already seen that professionals tend to hold a higher opinion of

---

*This statement is meant only as a general description. There certainly are many social service agencies that do have paraprofessionals in administrative decision-making roles; this is particularly true in agencies that grew out of the "self-help" rehabilitation movement.

research than do paraprofessionals. As a result an administrator may well have a more favorable view of the possible contributions of research to an agency's credibility than the agency's paraprofessional staff members. The consultant is thus likely to be called in by a professional from the ranks of administration and given a mandate to carry out research in an agency whose paraprofessional staff do not share the administrator's view of the importance of research.

The factors of "tradition" and "financial need" serve to solidify already existing differences between administration and paraprofessionals concerning the advantages of research consultants. The "tradition" factor works through the school system and tends to give administrators a relatively favorable attitude toward social research, and it tends to extend these positive attitudes into the realm where research may not have any direct relation to the effective operation of a service agency. Here we are dealing not with the usefulness of information already discovered, but with the potential advantage of research as a general approach to problem solving. Such a belief encourages administrators to look to researchers even in cases where research (or evaluation) is not a clear path to a solution of problems involving agency effectiveness, credibility, or financing. Here too we have a dynamic that tends to increase the differential between the willingness of degreed administrators and paraprofessional staff to tolerate the demands of research and evaluation consultants.

Financial pressure. Although continued funding is a concern of all of an agency's employees, it is the immediate responsibility of administrators, who are most likely to seek all possible methods of increasing an organization's credibility. As a result of such responsibility the differential acceptance of the consultant is further entrenched because the competent administrator is likely to seek out and employ all possible methods of showing the world that his organization is performing important and useful tasks. Moreover, administrators are likely to perceive involvement in research as worthwhile in and of itself and that involvement with research is a secondary activity that an agency can claim to its credit.

We are not dealing with a case of unconditional acceptance of research by administrators and unconditional rejection of research by other members of a service agency. The issue is one of the differential acceptance of research stemming from the administrator's responsibility to ensure the viability of an organization. Matters are made more difficult when paraprofessionals are involved because paraprofessional service delivery personnel tend to have particularly negative opinions about the value of research and evaluation. The factor of "administrator responsibility" operates even in cases where both administrators and service delivery personnel are paraprofessionals. The amount of the differential, however, and the extent to which "mutual need," "tradition," and "financial pressure" reinforce each other will depend to some extent on the professional and paraprofessional backgrounds of the administrators.

Methods for Easing Friction Between Paraprofessional Service Personnel and Research Consultants

The frictions that exist involve a complex interplay of psychological, sociologic, and historical factors. Many of the reasons for conflict are not only perfectly legitimate but also are grounded in the structure of the research and service systems; they cannot be completely solved without a radical (and probably undesirable) restructuring of present methods of social research and social service. [For an outline of the form that a constructive restructuring must take, see Morell (1975).] One can, however, enumerate certain steps that a researcher can take to alleviate or avoid at least some of the problems that might arise.

Dislocation in routine caused by research. It is the exceptional research project that does not get in the way of established routine. [For examples of research that is unobtrusive, see the work by Webb et al. (1966) and Hyman (1972).] The real problem arises when research is perceived not only as disruptive but also as not worthwhile or not legitimate. Consultants must try hard to keep their demands on staff to a minimum. Researchers have a strong tendency to try to collect all the information they can "just in case" it might be useful; this tendency must be resisted. A datum should not be collected unless there is good reason to believe that it is important and useful. (A side benefit might be more hypothesis testing and less post hoc analysis. The cause of social science would be well served if researchers' initial attitudes were that data are expensive, difficult to collect, and of dubious benefit to the questions being studied.) Furthermore, the consultant must try to communicate the message that every attempt is being made to keep research demands at a minimum and to explain to paraprofessional staff why any given demand for time or effort is really necessary.

Demystifying research. There is a mystique to the conduct of research that can easily be interpreted (rightly or wrongly) as arrogance on the part of the researcher. The mystique is a combination of the consultant's prestige, method of entry into the organization, esoteric methodology, and status as possessor of knowledge that is special, powerful, and important. The only way to remove this mystique is to explain what one is doing, and why.

Consultants must develop the attitude that research can be explained to the layman and that such explanations are worth the effort. The feasibility of such explanations has often been demonstrated by the numerous books and articles in all fields of science written for the specific purpose of explaining technical matters to laymen.

Such explanations are important because service delivery personnel very often serve the consultant by filling the role of data collector. Moreover, data collection often involves work that is not perceived as a normal part of one's job, for which there is no extra pay, and involving extra work. People who find themselves in such situations have a right to demand, at the very least, an understandable explanation of what they are involved in and why their services are needed. While it is certainly not true that all service personnel feel this way, consultants are likely to find many cases where the attitude of service delivery personnel is a serious impediment to research and evaluation. The only way to avoid such impediments is for the consultant to start every project with the attitude that agency personnel have a right to know and understand the significance of the demands made upon them.

Respect for the abilities of paraprofessionals. In large measures paraprofessional service personnel serve the consultant as experts without whose help research cannot be conducted. This position derives from the unique ability of many paraprofessionals to relate to a particular population, to obtain information from them, and to make judgements about them (Glasscote, Sussex, Jaffe, Ball, & Brill, 1972; Truax & Carkhuff, 1967). It seems not only counterproductive but also wrong for professional consultants to treat paraprofessionals in a manner that fails to convey a sense of the paraprofessionals' unique abilities and expertise.

Evaluation apprehension. Fear of being evaluated is always present when outsiders are allowed to view one's work; this is especially true in the case of paraprofessionals who work in social service. Funding for social service is always tenuous, and of all social service personnel paraprofessionals are most restricted in their job mobility potential (Morell, 1975). A consultant conducting an evaluation can do little to alleviate the tension inherent in the situation. (The assurance that programs and not personnel are being evaluated may be true but serves as small consolation.) The only recourse that the consultant has is to take the needs of the agency into account and to evaluate the agency on criteria that it can legitimately and reasonably be expected to meet.

The issue of legitimate and reasonable criteria are important because agency personnel have good reason to believe that evaluators expect too much of social service agencies. Etzioni (1969) claims that organizations must split their efforts between organizational maintenance and stated objectives.

It follows that a social unit that devotes all its efforts to fulfilling one functional requirement, even if it is that of performing goal activities, will undermine the fulfillment of this very functional requirement, because recruitment of means, maintenance of tools, and the social integration of the unit will be neglected.

He further claims that evaluators tend to look only at stated goals and to carry out their evaluations with the implicit assumption that stated goals are the only legitimate objectives of an organization.

According to Campbell (1971) any advocacy, by its nature, must involve exaggerated and inflated claims. If there is any truth to this, and if we assume that employees of an agency are also advocates of the goals of the agency, the reasons for evaluation apprehension become clear. Nobody wants to be forced into the position of defending the proposition that an agency is a failure unless it meets its overtly stated, exaggerated objectives. Furthermore, there are reasons to believe that the impact of many social agencies will, of necessity, be small. Rossi (1972) argues

. . . similarly with respect to our social ills. Dramatic effects on illiteracy can be achieved by providing schools and teachers to all children. Achieving a universally high enough level of literacy and knowledge, so that everyone capable of learning can find a good spot in our labor force, is a bit more difficult. Hence the more we have done in the past to lower unemployment rates, to provide social services, etc., the more difficult it is to add to the benefits derived from past programs by the addition of new ones. Partly, this is because we have achieved so much with the past programs and partly this is because the massive efforts of the past have not dealt with individual motivation as much as with the benefits to aggregates of individuals.*

According to Weiss (1970),

Fragmentary projects are created to deal with broad-spectrum problems. We know about multiple causality. We realize that a single stimulus program is hardly likely to make a dent in deep rooted ills. But the political realities are such that we take what programs can get through Congress (and other sources) when we can get them.

Although most social service personnel cannot present arguments as clearly as these, it is very likely that they have a feeling for these issues and that their fear of evaluation is based on these arguments.

The evaluator must not only take these matters into account when designing evaluation but must also go out of his way to make sure that the staff he is evaluating is aware of his concern for such issues.** Evaluation apprehension

*From Rossi, P.H. Boobytraps and pitfalls in the evaluation of social action programs. In C. Weiss (Ed.), *Evaluating action programs: Readings in social action research*. Boston: Allyn and Bacon, 1972.

**For an excellent discussion of evaluation research techniques, see the works of Isaac (1974), Moursund (1973), Suchman (1967), Tripodi, Fellin, & Epstein (1973), and Riecken & Boruch (1974).

is serious enough in any evaluative situation. It is even more of a problem
when a consultant has to deal with paraprofessionals, who of all service
agency employees have the least professional credibility and therefore the
most to lose if an agency's funding is lowered.

Usefulness of research and the consultant's credibility. Many researchers feel that unless they claim that their work has practical significance they
will not be given the resources or the opportunity to conduct the research that
interests them. In this age of tight funding and restricted budgets, research is
often regarded as a dispensible frill. A consequence of this attitude is that
researchers often grasp at any possible argument, no matter how tenuous, to
justify their work. To make matters worse, it is quite likely that many researchers have grown to believe their own propaganda in this matter. The
result is a loss of credibility for researchers that is particularly serious among
paraprofessionals, who generally tend to have a low regard for the benefits of
science and research.

The only way to solve this problem is for research consultants to be
scrupulously careful about any claims they might make. The problem of
unmet expectations will not arise if the true value of the work is known to
agency personnel from the start. The value of any given research project
cannot, of course, be accurately predicted. The question of whether or not
research will be used for practical purposes involves sociologic matters that
transcend issues of validity or reliability or theoretical implications of the
work. It is equally true, however, that intelligent guesses of why a given piece
of research is worthwhile can also be made. Researchers have tended to inflate
these estimates, with the result that their credibility has decreased in the eyes
of those who do not start out with strong beliefs in the value of research.

Authority of consultant. Although research may be accepted by the
administrators of an agency, it may not be welcomed. (This is particularly true
when we are talking about evaluation.) If administrators accept a consultant
only half-heartedly at a time when other staff have even more negative feelings about the consultant, there is little hope for successful research. This
situation can easily be made even worse if the rights of the consultant have not
been clarified before the start of a project. How much time is the consultant
allowed to demand of an agency's staff? What effort can the consultant
demand of service agency personnel? What information can the consultant ask
for? These and numerous similar questions can result in endless quarreling
between consultant and agency staff. The best solution is for the consultant to
clarify these matters at the outset, to communicate his expectations to all
involved, and to insist that the agency's administrators back him up when he

begins to ask staff for time and effort. [An interesting discussion of the contents of negotiations between researchers and agency administrators can be found in a report by Fairweather, Sanders, & Tornatzky (1974).]

It is clear that heeding these warnings and following this advice cannot by itself guarantee smooth relations between a research consultant and the paraprofessional staff of a social agency. The advice was presented in the hope that it will sensitize the reader to problems that might arise and that it might point to a direction for amelioration of problems when they do arise.

CONCLUSIONS

In sum, this chapter presented a general analysis of the issues involved in contact between consultants and paraprofessionals in the field of social service. It concluded that most such contacts take place either in the context of in-service training or in the context of research and evaluation. It further concluded that in each of these contexts there are crucial issues that are independent of the specific content of any given training or research program and that the consultant must be aware of these general issues in order to render quality service to social service agencies which are staffed by paraprofessionals.

REFERENCES

Albee, G. W. Models, myths and manpower. *Mental Hygiene,* 1968, *52,* 168–180.

Andrade, S. J., & Burstein, A. G. Social congruence and empathy in paraprofessional mental health workers. *Community Mental Health Journal,* 1973, *9,* 388–397.

Aronson, S. H., & Sherwood, C. C. Researcher versus practitioner: Problems in social action research. *Social Work,* 1967, *12,* 89–96.

Bergen, B. J. Professional communities and the evaluation of demonstration projects in community mental health. In H. C. Schulberg, A. Sheldon, & F. Baker, (Eds.), *Program evaluation in the health fields.* New York: Behavioral Publications, 1969.

Bloom, B. C. Mental health program evaluation. In S. E. Golann, & C. Eisdorfer, (Eds.), *Handbook of community mental health.* New York: Appleton-Century-Crofts, 1972.

Caro, F. G. Evaluation research—An overview. In F. G. Caro, (Ed.), *Readings in evaluation research.* New York: Russell Sage Foundation, 1971.

Cooper, S. Role diffusions—Dilemmas and problems. In H. Guttesfeld (Ed.), *The critical issues of community mental health.* New York: Behavioral Publications, 1972.

Cowen, E. L., & Zax, M. The mental health field today: Issues and problems. In E. L. Cowen, E. A. Gardner, & M. Zax, (Eds.), *Emergent approaches to mental health problems.* New York: Appleton-Century-Crofts, 1967.

Etzioni, A. Two approaches to organizational analysis: A critique and a suggestion. In
    H. C. Schulberg, A. Sheldon, & F. Baker, (Eds.), *Program evaluation in the
    health fields.* New York: Behavioral Publications, 1969.

Fairweather, G. W. *Methods for experimental social innovation.* New York: Wiley,
    1967.

Fairweather, G. W., Sanders, D. H., & Tornatzky, L. G. *Creating change in mental
    health organizations.* New York: Pergamon, 1974.

Fringe, J. Research and the service agency. *Social Casework,* 1952, *33,* 343–348.

Glasscote, R. M., Sussex, J. N., Jaffe, J. H., Ball, J., & Brill, L. *The treatment of
    drug abuse: Programs, problems, prospects.* American Psychiatric Association,
    Washington, D. C., 1974.

Howard, K. I., & Orlinsky, D. E. Psychotherapeutic progress. *Annual Review of
    Psychology,* 1972, *23,* 615–668.

Hyman, H. H. *Secondary analysis of sample surveys: Principles and potentialities.*
    New York: Wiley, 1972.

Isaac, S., & Michael, W. B. *Handbook in research and evaluation for education and
    the behavioral sciences.* San Diego: Edits Publishing Company, 1977.

Karlsruher, A. E. The nonprofessional as a psychotherapeutic agent. *American Jour-
    nal of Community Psychology,* 1974, *2,* 61–77.

Kuhn, T. S. *The structure of scientific revolutions.* Chicago: University of Chicago
    Press, 1970.

Lakatos, I., & Musgrave, A. (Eds.) *Criticism and the growth of knowledge.* London,
    New York: Cambridge University Press, 1970.

Levin, J. One road to survival—Alternate education for the non-degreed substance
    abuse worker. *Proceedings of the 7th Annual Eagleville Conference,* June 5–7,
    1974, Eagleville, Pa. Published by Alcohol, Drug Abuse and Mental Health
    Administration (DHEW Publication No. ADM 75–227), 1975.

Lipsey, M. W. Research and relevance: A survey of graduate students and faculty in
    psychology. *American Psychologist,* 1974, *29,* 541–553.

Mann, J. *Changing human behavior.* New York: Scribners, 1965.

Meltzoff, J., & Kornreich, M. *Research in psychotherapy.* New York: Atherton,
    1970.

Morell, J. A. Blocks to job mobility for paraprofessionals in community based re-
    habilitation programs. Paper presented to the American Public Health Associa-
    tion, November 16–20, 1975, Chicago, Illinois.

Morell, J. A. The conflict between research and mental health services. *Administration
    in Mental Health.* Spring, 1977, 52–58.

Moursund, J. P. *Evaluation: An introduction to research design.* Monterey, Cal.:
    Brooks-Cole Publishing Company, 1973.

National Task Force On The Continuing Education Unit. *The Continuing Education
    Unit: Criteria and Guidelines.* Washington, D.C.: National University Extension
    Association, 1974.

Ottenberg, D. J. Traditional and nontraditional credentials in addictive problems—A
    dispatch from the battlefield. *Proceedings of the 7th Annual Eagleville Confer-
    ence,* June 5–7, 1974, Eagleville, Pa. Published by Alcohol, Drug Abuse and
    Mental Health Administration (DHEW Publication No. ADM 75-227), 1975.

Peth, P. A critical examination of the role and function of the non-professional in rehabilitation. *Rehabilitation and Counseling Bulletin*, 1971, *14*, 141−151.

Rein, G. Alliances of professionals and paraprofessionals: Who owns the turf? *Hospital and Community Psychiatry*, 1975, *26*, 759−760.

Riecken, H. W., & Boruch, R. F. (Eds.) *Social experimentation: A method for planning and evaluating social intervention*. New York: Academic Press, 1974.

Rimm, D. C., & Masters, J. L. *Behavior therapy–Techniques and empirical findings*. New York: Academic Press, 1974.

Rodman, H., & Kolodny, R. Organizational strains in the researcher−practitioner relationship. *Human Organization*, 1964, *23*, 171−182.

Rossi, P. H. Boobytraps and pitfalls in the evaluation of social action programs. In C. Weiss, (Eds.), *Evaluating action programs: Readings in social action research*. Boston: Allyn and Bacon, 1972.

Siegel, J. S. Mental health volunteers as change agents. *American Journal of Community Psychology*, 1973, *7*, 138−158.

Sparer, G. O.E.O. drug treatment programs: Are community-based non-professional drug free programs effective? *Public Health Reports*, 1975, *90*, 455-459.

Suchmann, E. A. *Evaluative research*. New York: Russell Sage Foundation, 1967.

Suinn, B. M. Traits for selection of paraprofessionals for behavior-modification consultation training. *Community Mental Health Journal*, 1974, *10*, 441−449.

Tripodi, T., Epstein, I., & Fellin, P. *Social program evaluation: Guidelines for Health, Education and Welfare administrators*. Itasca, Illinois: Peacock Publishers, 1971.

Truax, C. B., & Carkhuff, R. R. *Toward effective counseling and psychotherapy*. Chicago: Aldine, 1967.

Truax, C. B., & Mitchell, K. M. Research on certain therapist interpersonal skills in relation to process and outcome. In A. E. Bergin & S. L. Garfield (Eds.), *Handbook of psychotherapy and behavior change: An empirical analysis*. New York: Wiley, 1971.

Webb, E., Campbell, D. T., Schwartz, R., & Sechrest, L. *Unobstrusive measures: Nonreactive research in the social sciences*. New York: Rand-McNally, 1966.

Weiss, C. H. The politicization of evaluation research. *Journal of Social Issues*, 1970, *26*, 57−68.

Wolman, B. B. *Handbook of clinical psychology*. New York: McGraw-Hill, 1965.

Thomas D. Cook,
Alphonse Buccino

5

The Social Scientist as a Provider of Consulting Services to the Federal Government

In a memorandum to the heads of executive departments and agencies dated May 12, 1977, President Carter wrote:

In a continuing search for ways to improve the efficiency and effectiveness of the executive branch, I have become aware of a need for improved management of the excessively large volume of consulting and expert services used by the Federal Government. A recent survey by a Senate subcommittee of the use of personal and nonpersonal consultant and expert services, identified more than 30,000 contract arrangements and 10,777 individual appointments. Additionally, there are such services provided by grant arrangements and through advisory committee memberships.

There has been, and continues to be, evidence that some consulting services, including experts and advisors are being used excessively, unnecessarily, and improperly.

Also in 1977, the Subcommittee on Reports, Accounting, and Management of the Committee on Governmental Affairs of the United States Senate issued a 610-page report on ''Consultants and Contractors.'' The chairman, the late Senator Metcalf, wrote:

During recent years, growing sums of money have been spent on increasing numbers of Federal consultants and contractors for a widening array of services. No

The views expressed are those of the authors and do not necessarily reflect those of the National Science Foundation.

The authors wish to thank Robert Boruch, Robert B. Hardy, Larry C. Kerpelman, George J. Lynch, and Allen M. Shinn, Jr. for their perceptive comments on previous drafts of this paper.

one has been able to say with certainty how many (consultants and contractors) there are, who they are, or how much we spend on their services. (p. 1)

Both President Carter and the U.S. Senate Subcommittee on Reports, Accounting, and Management, Committee on Governmental Affairs have noted that the Federal government uses too many consultants and contractors and that the usage is increasing. Our purpose is to discuss why the number of consultants has been increasing, why there is disaffection with consultants and contractors, and how the consultants and contractors might be better employed for achieving the purposes of the Federal government. To meet these goals, we shall have to define "consultant" and "contractor" and describe both the tasks they perform and the processes by which they are selected and managed by Federal officials.

Our explicit concern is with consulting services offered by social scientists employed by universities and contract research firms. These persons are usually trained in economics, sociology, political science, education, psychology, business, social work, or related disciplines. They are a minority of all consultants, since the Federal government makes extensive use of natural scientists, of managers from private industry and labor organizations, and of representatives of professional groups and civic societies as well as many other kinds of persons.

DEFINITIONS

In its colloquial usage, the term *consultant* is usually understood to mean someone who gives professional advice or services regarding matters in the field of that person's special knowledge when asked to do so by an agency. Consultants are hired by the Federal government in three principal contexts.

The first context occurs when an agency solicits advice or other services from an individual who operates alone (*individual consultation*). Some consultation of this kind is done by university faculty members, often from better-known institutions. Frequently the statement of work to be performed is quite brief, and often no written product is expected from the consultant's services.

The second context occurs when an agency solicits advice from individuals as members of an advisory panel (*advisory committee consultation*). The Federal Government uses committees to obtain advice and recommendations regarding—among other things—which directions an agency's programs might take, how a program or particularly important project is progressing, and which grant proposals should be funded. Such consultation is carried out by well-known experts or by representatives of organizations with a special competence or interest in the topic on which advice is requested.*

It is clear from President Carter's memorandum and the Subcommittee report that their concerns extend beyond the use of consultants in the senses above. They also include a concern with contractors, profit-making or not-for-profit companies that agree by contract to perform designated services for the Federal Government. Contractors might be thought of as consultants who work in companies, but technically the government purchases services from the company and not from individuals in the company. Many companies exist to provide such service, including such well-known organizations as Arthur D. Little, Rand Corporation, Educational Testing Service, ABT Associates, Stanford Research Institute, Booz, Allen, & Hamilton, Ernst & Ernst, and Westinghouse. Numerous small firms also exist, and the Washington, D.C. telephone directory lists hundreds of organizations offering social science and management expertise, almost always to the Federal Government; some of these firms have only one or two professionals.

The distinction between contractors, who offer services from research firms that depend on contracts for their existence, and consultants, who offer services but do not work directly for such firms, is a working distinction that has often been used, as it was in the Metcalf subcommittee report. However, the distinction is not always preserved in public discussions. For instance, a headline in the *Chicago Tribune* of Sunday, May 8, 1977, read "U.S. Consults Consultants About Consultants," and the article dealt with the fact that HEW had issued a contract to Rockwell International to discover how many consultants HEW had hired from private industry. Moreover, the distinction is difficult to maintain at a more formal level in that some consultants are reimbursed for their services by means of a "personal services contract," while the employees of some contract research companies serve as individual consultants to the government and other research firms.

However, we find it convenient to use the terminology of the Office of Management and Budget (OMB), which refers to "consulting services," including "personal and professional services of a purely advisory nature relating to the development of agency policy . . . *provided by persons and / or firms* . . . who are generally considered to have knowledge and ability distinctively valuable to the agency" (Federal Register, Vol. 42, December 16, 1977, p. 63492) [italics added]. Here individual consultants and contract research firms are clearly similar in that each provides "consultant services," a similarity further highlighted when in the same document ser-

---

*Both individual and advisory panel consultation are sometimes provided for in research grants or contracts, in which case individuals need not be directly solicited by Federal officials, although they sometimes need to be approved by them.

vices are outlined that exemplify consultant services, including both services predominantly conducted by contract research firms (e.g., analysis of the impact of programs; policy and program analysis evaluation and advice) and services conducted by advisory panels (e.g., grant peer review panels). While we have chosen not always to preserve the distinction between consultants and contractors, there is one respect in which the distinction is important: Government use of individual consultants is regulated by the Federal Personnel System, while contracting is regulated by Federal Procurement Regulations. Members of formal Advisory Committees usually are appointed as individual consultants, but Committee and agency uses of them are also subject to the Federal Advisory Committee Act (Public Law 92-463).

WHO OFFERS CONSULTING SERVICES, AND WHAT TASKS DO THEY PERFORM?

Individual Consultation

Individual consultants are frequently used on an ad hoc basis for discussion and advice about what a Federal official or office should do, how things should be done, or how reports should be evaluated. The consultant's contribution is supposed to help Federal officials keep apprised of the current state of the art in important substantive and methodological areas and to help officials gain fresh perspectives about the tasks they have to perform.

The criteria for selecting individual consultants differ with the task to be performed and the thoroughness with which selection is made, but the criteria can include evaluating the prospective consultant's (1) level of expertise or experience, as indexed by a curriculum vitae or an opinion from a respected person, (2) flexibility and willingness to consider multiple perspectives on how an issue should be defined or how action should be taken, (3) ability to be as objective as possible or to represent a biased point of view known to complement that of some other consultant, (4) past history of doing the necessary reading of documents and reports in preparation for a meeting, (5) ability to perform promised work in timely fashion, (6) tact and discretion, (7) willingness to make special efforts on the agency's behalf when special efforts are required, and (8) degree of connection in a well-known network of persons who have demonstrated intellectual expertise or political power in the substantive matters of relevance. It is rare that all of these criteria are used in selecting a consultant; even when a particular selection criterion is especially important, it is rare to find a thorough search for information about this criterion. A few questions to a few colleagues may be all the information search that takes place.

The selection of consultants depends heavily on informal connections between Federal officials and members of both the scientific community and other Federal agencies. Consequently, several mechanisms have evolved to try to limit "cronyism" and weed out incompetence. First, agencies must follow internal approval procedures in appointing a new consultant; these include obtaining approval from senior members of the agency. Second, agencies must make a positive effort to reappoint consultants, since their term of appointment automatically lapses after a fixed time period (usually one year). It therefore is not easy to have a friend appointed as a consultant and kept in that status in the face of poor performing. Third, in many instances consultants interact with more members of an agency than the person who invited them, and they often produce reports that are read by several persons other than the one who made the appointment. Few agency officials will reappoint a consultant whose mannerisms or skills—to the extent that they can be evaluated—could embarrass them.

Individual consultants perform a wide variety of tasks, from helping administrators conceptualize new directions for their agencies through reviewing and advising on questionnaires or first drafts of final reports. Usually the skills tapped include background knowledge of particular theories relevant to the mandate of a particular agency or knowledge of the technical skills required to implement particular projects. One other form of knowledge on the part of consultants is worth stressing. Young persons most often come to the attention of Federal officials as prospective consultants when well-known persons are invited to consult on a particular issue but cannot and suggest other names, including the names of their proteges or of up-and-coming scholars they know or have heard about.

Kelling (1977) has provided an interesting commentary on what consultants can do well, at least in evaluation research, and we present his thoughts here in some detail. Three critical points stand out concerning what they can do:

(a) "Now that I have all this data, why did I collect it in the first place and what should I do with it?" In other words, it is possible that the evaluator will get so immersed in detail that he will forget what the original goals of the project were and how the data [deal] with those goals. Further, after being removed from the world of academia during a year or two of the evaluation, the evaluator may need some assistance in updating his/her statistical skills. The consultant or consultants can help the field staff of an evaluation to review their work and update skills.

(b) Review the outline for the presentation of the findings. This is related to 'a' and is a part of 'a' that is so important that I separated it out. Getting a good outline of the final report is *the* critical issue in getting the evaluator to put his/her pen to paper. It nicely makes a completely unmanageable task (completing the report) into a manageable one.

(c) Finally—reading the preliminary draft of the evaluation and providing con-structive, non-threatening advice. Generally upon completing the first draft, the evaluator thinks (hopes) that he/she is finished writing. In fact, he/she has just begun. Remember, *any* first draft, regardless of its weaknesses, is good. If an evaluator is reasonably good and has good consultation, *any* first draft almost assures completion.

So much for the positive contributions of consultants. They can make real and substantial contributions, but for all parties involved in the conduct of an evaluation, it is certainly best to underestimate their contributions rather than to overestimate them.

They *cannot:*

1. Supervise staff. Young, energetic staff need constant and ongoing stroking, direction, love and supervision. Consultants cannot provide that. They do not have the time, nor do they control the means and rewards necessary to manage staff.

2. Develop evaluation instruments (questionnaires, etc.). Instruments must be developed by resident evaluation staff in close collaboration with agency program staff. Consultants don't have the time, energy, and generally, the patience to collaborate as closely as necessary.

3. Write up results. The writing of the final report is a consuming full-time task. Consultants are involved in too many things to be expected to write up a final report.

The key thing to remember in dealing with consultants (and I do not mean this critically) is that they are *un*responsible. They are bright, knowledgeable, clever, but they have no responsibility for the final product and rarely, if ever, will be cornered into accepting such responsibility. They have different responsibilities and will meet those first—that is to be expected. Neither the program evaluator [nor] administration should be surprised by this as likely they, too, are consultants some place.

Advisory Committee Consultation

It is useful to distinguish between advisory committees selected for tech-nical expertise and those selected because a variety of different viewpoints must be represented. The first type of committee is exemplified by cases where an agency appoints several persons to monitor a particularly important but difficult research project or to report on how a research area is likely to develop in the next ten years. The second type is exemplified by, say, the Review Panel on Labs and Centers of the National Institute of Education (NIE), a committee composed of scholars, school administrators, school prin-cipals, and citizens from many cultural backgrounds and many parts of the country.*

*While the distinction between technical and heterogeneous boards is quite easy to make in practice, it is difficult to justify in the abstract because a technical panel on new research directions—say, in physics—would usually be chosen to reflect the known heterogeneity among physicists. Even when the panel is concerned with a narrower area—e.g., high-energy particle

Several functions of committees beside giving advice can be distinguished. Often the committees are empowered to make formal recommendations about policy. Indeed, the committee members are usually chosen so as to increase the credibility and legitimacy of any advice or recommendations that come from them, irrespective of whether the recommendations deal with research proposals that should be funded, directions that future research should take, or roles science should play in society. Legitimacy is conferred because the committee's advice is believed to reflect a consensus reached after long and informed deliberation. The underlying model can be characterized as: "balance through the representation of multiple acceptable viewpoints"; thus persons holding extreme viewpoints are probably not often appointed to committees. Sometimes the committee's formal function is to provide "oversight" (e.g., to review the progress on an important research project or to assess the degree of compliance with some regulation). In this case, the committee members try to improve the efficiency of the project being overseen by motivating operators to perform better and by providing practical hints about how things can be improved.*

The process for selecting advisory committees, unlike that for individual consultants, is almost always formal. The first step (as provided by the Federal Advisory Committee Act) is filing a charter and obtaining approval of the Office of Management and Budget to establish the committee. The next step usually is to canvass qualified people recognized by the agency in order to generate a wide range of nominations. With heterogeneous committees a range of skills, vested interests, and distributional characteristics (e.g., geography, age, race, sex) is deliberately sought. For technical committees, skills are much more important than distributional requirements, and distributional requirements are usually more important than a balance of vested interests. Nonetheless, skill is rarely the *sole* criterion. The next step is to select from the nominees those individuals who represent an agency-determined balance. Sometimes—but increasingly rarely—veto rights are given to interest groups at this stage, as happened when scholars whose research indicated that television might be harmful to children were excluded from the Surgeon General's Committee on Television and Violence at the request of the television industry (Cater & Strickland, 1975). After the committee is selected, deliberation and report writing follow.

---

physics—there will still be heterogeneity among such physicists. Such variability seems small, though, relative to that found in a board set up to reflect multiple competencies, including different professions and/or different interest groups and perhaps even the general public.

*Other functions of boards could be listed, including those of lending prestige to an agency by virtue of the individual reputations of board members and even obeying the law because a formal regulation requires that a board be set up.

Technical advisory committees are normally composed of prominent people in the substantive area of concern, many of whose names will be known to Federal officials before the nominating process begins. Even so the nominating process will result in some new names, particularly if distributional requirements of geography, race, sex, or subdisciplines are needed. Heterogeneous advisory committees usually include formal representatives of specific constituency groups, and the choice of the individual board member is frequently left to the group itself. This situation often gives rise to the appearance of conflict of interest, since it appears that groups with vested interests are asked to nominate persons to advise the government, although the advice they give supposedly comes from an independent committee. Where no organized constituency exists, or where the agency feels it should not approach the formal constituency group, someone will be chosen whose personal attributes include those that define the relevant group (e.g., "consumer," "female psychologist").

The criteria by which selection is made, and the quality control mechanisms that officials can use, are more formalized than those previously listed for individual consultants. A major difference is that with heterogeneous committees political considerations of "representativeness" and "balance" are extremely important. Indeed, Federal officials must be prepared to tolerate some tactlessness and irresponsibility from committee members who fail to attend meetings or do not read prepared documents carefully, since terminating an appointment prematurely would lose "balance" or "representativeness."

The effectiveness of advisory boards is hard to assess, given their variability. However, Cook & Gruder (1978) claimed that such boards are often inefficient for gaining fresh insights into a problem and coming up with timely and realistic advice about how to improve performance. Timely and realistic advice is problematic once the board reaches a certain—but as yet unknown—size and degree of heterogeneity, suggesting that both technical and heterogeneous committees may function best to legitimize decisions that do not have to be made in haste.

Contractors

HOW CONTRACTORS ARE CHOSEN

Contract research differs from consulting in that the focus is more on the tasks to be performed than on an individual's special skills. The most relevant tasks for social scientists are needs analysis, policy analysis, and program evaluation. The contract research industry can best be thought of as the decentralized research arm of the government, performing tasks of information gathering and assimilation that in many other countries are carried out by direct employees of the national government.

Formal procedures have to be followed in establishing contracts. The first step is for the government to determine its requirements regarding the scope of work, period of performance, and so forth. A number of different routes may then be taken to get a contract in place, but the process perhaps most familiar to persons outside government involves writing a Request for Proposals (RFP) describing the service the Federal Government would like to have performed. A notice of this RFP is then published in the Commerce Business Daily (CBD), and the RFP is distributed to all who request it. Interested contract research firms or universities then write proposals to perform the work; after these have been reviewed an organization is awarded the contract.

RFPs differ tremendously in clarity and specificity both within and between agencies. Some are perfunctory, while others go into great detail about the definition of the research problem, the approach to be taken, the timing of the research, and the level of effort required at each stage. In such cases, very little is left to the potential bidder's discretion or professional judgment. Most RFPs are open to all bidders, but a few are restricted to bidders from minority groups or small businesses who might otherwise find it difficult to compete against the major applied research firms.

Nearly all proposals have to be submitted within one or two months of the RFP first appearing, which is not long for preparing a document that may be quite lengthy and technically complex. Hence most contract firms have techniques to speed the writing process. Some sections of a proposal (e.g., those dealing with management, company description, company capabilities) may be lifted ''off the shelf'' and used without modification. However, speed of response is usually achieved by efficiency of organization and smoothness of procedures in evaluating an RFP, deciding to respond, writing the technical plan, and preparing cost estimates. When necessary, many persons will work on a proposal simultaneously.

Both the considerable incentive to submit proposals and the short time interval allotted for the proposal submission have caused contract research firms to cultivate arrangements that lead to early warnings about the topics of new RFPs, about possible appearance dates, and about how much the research might be worth. Informal contacts with individuals in agencies are most likely to produce such information, which allows extra time for proposal writing and for developing a relationship with the person who might later monitor the contract. While it is illegal for agency employees to talk about procurements that have already been published in the CBD and about specific RFPs being planned, it is legal to talk in a general way about future agency plans and office or section responsibilities. It may help to have a former agency employee on the staff at the right time, but most contracting firms deal with so many agencies it is probably not possible to cultivate a systematic advantage in this way.

The process of contractor selection involves formal review of all proposals. The review is usually performed by employees of the agency letting the contract, to whom the final report will be furnished. The major criterion for funding a proposal is its technical adequacy in meeting goals of the RFP at a reasonable cost, but organizational capability also plays a role. Selection can be made following initial review, but it is not uncommon (especially for larger and more complex contracts) for the initial review to identify a set of "technically acceptable" or "competitive" proposals. When this is done, the remaining competitors usually have an opportunity to revise their technical proposals in the light of reviewer comments and submit best-and-final offers. Even after this stage there may be extensive negotiations to establish more precisely what work is to be done and the appropriate cost.

WHO GETS THE CONTRACTS

Most of the dollars for contract research by social scientists go to a dozen or so firms (some of which were listed earlier) that have traditionally received many of the contracts for large surveys, experiments, and evaluations. These firms employ scores of professionals from most of the social science disciplines, although some firms may be better noted for their work in education than economics or vice versa. Backing up these professionals with advanced degrees is a staff that helps with proposals and with reports, the collections and analysis of data, the management of fiscal matters, and the upkeep of buildings. Some of the firms have issued stock and are profit making; others are not-for-profit and charge a fee over and above the research costs and overhead to stimulate growth and development in much the same way as profits. There is therefore little practical distinction between profit and not-for-profit companies.

Although the large firms are more capable of carrying out large contracts, this is not the case with moderate or small contracts. (We shall arbitrarily assume that contracts in excess of $150,000 per annum are large, those between $149,999 and $50,000 are moderate, and those less than $50,000 are small.) Large contract research firms bid for moderate-sized contracts, which give them a chance to earn money and build agency contracts and which also provide an outlet for the entrepreneurial zeal of individual principal investigators within these firms. The large firms are less likely to bid for small contracts, particularly short-term ones, since the competition is fiercer and the financial return will hardly justify the expense of proposal writing. Even so, proposals for smaller contracts are still made by some persons from such firms who work on several small contracts simultaneously.

The smaller firms that bid for moderate and small contracts differ enormously, from companies with up to a dozen professionals and a solid record of accomplishments to companies with a single professional and little or no record of completed work. Most of the very small firms are located in the Washington, D.C. area and are nothing more than individual consultants who have left a large contract research firm or a government agency in the hope of establishing themselves. Many of these smaller companies stay in business for just a short period and then either die out or emerge later under a different name. They usually respond to many RFPs in a year, since they are at a disadvantage compared to large firms because funding decisions are made partly on the basis of organizational capability to perform the research and/or the experience and training of the researchers. A hope of many small contractors is to bid for a contract on which no one else bids, or at least to bid for a contract on which no one from the major companies bids. They are helped here because agencies often set aside funds for small business. While some small firms occasionally offer special capabilities that aid them in obtaining large contracts, it seems to us that large contracts usually go to the larger contract research firms.

There are many reasons why universities have not often bid for contracts in the past, especially large ones: (1) most contracts require interdisciplinary cooperation, and universities are organized along disciplinary lines; (2) most academics have to perform tasks irrelevant to completing a contract (e.g., teaching or publishing); (3) contracts usually contain clauses limiting publication of the results and data ownership, and decisions about research procedures are ultimately in the hands of Federal officials and not researchers; (4) the quick response time to RFPs usually prevents faculty members from bidding, since they may have difficulty freeing time on short notice for proposal preparation because of unbreakable teaching and research obligations; and (5) even if they are awarded a large contract, many universities may have difficulty in finding staff to do the research, from keypunch operators to data collectors to data processors and technical writers. Although these factors limit university involvement in contract research, they do not eliminate it entirely, particularly for stable, large research centers. Moreover, it is our impression that more and more universities are trying to develop an organizational capability for contract bidding. If so, some of the limitations mentioned above may be corrected by universities in the near future.

CONTRACTOR ACTIVITIES INSIDE FIRMS

Most of the time of middle-level or starting professionals is spent simply working on projects in technical capacities appropriate to their skills. People with doctorates or advanced professional degrees (MBA, MPH, etc.) who may have leadership roles will also spend time on administrative aspects of the contracts they have won. Professionals are responsible for the quality and timeliness of reports; to accomplish this they must make sure their staffs understand their responsibilities, their deadlines, and how much of their time is owed to the contract. (A staff member may work on a number of projects simultaneously.) Where field work is involved, professionals are also responsible for liaison with field personnel, whether the principals or superintendents of local schools or their own field staffs at a particular site. The professional is also responsible within his own firm for spending research funds wisely and within budget in a manner commensurate with the firm's fiscal policies. Additionally, the professional is responsible for the technical quality of reports and for obtaining any needed help from consultants or other staff of the firm. Finally, the professional must function as the liaison with the technical contract monitor from the sponsoring Federal agency, the person responsible for seeing that the technical (i.e., nonfiscal) aspects of the contract are carried out. Much of a professional's time with a monitor is spent justifying proposed actions or explaining interim reports. This contact with the government project officer usually occurs at all stages of the work, since the contract manager does not want to be in the position of having developed something that, later on, the project officer ultimately does not like or want.

The balance among technical, administrative, and management duties may be quite variable depending on the size of the firm, the size and complexity of the project, and management practices. For example, some contracting firms designate a senior management official (perhaps a vice-president) as responsible for each contract. While such an official's time on a given project may be small, the official does relieve the other substantive professionals of some management responsibilities.

In addition to administration and research, a professional in a contract research firm must spend some time raising money through new contracts; this involves scanning the CBD, obtaining RFPs, deciding which ones to bid on, and maintaining contacts with agencies to track priorities. Related to this, professionals may also spend some time selling their talents internally in order to get their own times up to 100 percent billable to contracts.

Generally speaking, a professional in a contract research firm has less opportunity than, say, a faculty member of developing independence to do research as one pleases. An exception might be senior professionals with well-established intellectual reputations. Similarly, publishing in professional journals and presenting papers at conferences and conventions is a more minor part of the contract researcher's role; indeed, it is probably of no importance to the smaller and moderately sized firms. In general, it is only the larger contract research firms that foster publishing, although usually as a lower priority than obtaining contracts and doing the resulting research. Given that it does not interfere with the higher priority tasks, publishing is approved, since it helps with the firm's image, enhances the credibility of the investigator, and adds to the knowledge base.

WHY ARE CONSULTANT SERVICES USED SO HEAVILY BY THE FEDERAL GOVERNMENT?

The dependence on consulting services is obvious to anyone who has spent time in Washington or in regional offices of the Federal Government. It is difficult to estimate the dollar amount of consulting services, the number of consultants, and the way consulting services have been changing over the years. The problems in doing this are outlined in the study commissioned by the Metcalf subcommittee. They include defining terms, determining the communality of definitions across various agencies, and making sense of the different ways that agencies record the use of consultants, experts, contractors, and advisory boards. A very rough indication of the amount of consulting services to *all* the Federal Government is provided by Guttman & Willner (1976), who suggest that in 1946 the largest single portion of the Federal administrative budget—30 percent—was spent on the Civil Service payroll (i.e., regular bureaucrats), while by 1966, 34 percent of the administrative budget was spent on contractors and only 22 percent on full-time government employees. The percentage is probably considerably greater now than in 1966, since some Washington observers believe that the rate of increase has been most rapid in the last ten years. Just what the current level of expenditure is on *social science* consultants and how this has been changing over the years are not yet known, but we see no reason why it should be different from the trend for all consultants and may even be greater given recent emphasis on social action programs and research.

The Expanding Technical Role of Government

We are witnessing an ever-expanding role for the Federal Government and an increasing need for information to fulfill its role. In the early days of the republic the decennial census was a simple head-count to determine congressional districts. Later on, when the Government began to establish immigration quotas, the census was tied to race and ethnic data, which had to be collected with more care. Proper regulation of the Social Security program requires data regarding age and employment status. Establishment of fiscal policy and regulation of the economy through such things as interest rates requires information regarding money in circulation and business conditions. In response to these new tasks the Census Bureau now performs many sophisticated special analyses in addition to simple head-counts, and new agencies such as the Bureau of Labor Statistics and the Bureau of Economic Analysis have come into being.

An increasing demand for services as well as information is illustrated by the role of the Federal Government in education. A Department of Education was established in 1867 with responsibility for "collecting such statistics and facts as shall show the condition and progress of education in the several states and territories, and of diffusing such information respecting the organization and management of schools and school systems, the methods of teaching, as shall aid the people of the United States in the establishment and maintenance of efficient school systems. . . ." This mandate hardly changed until 1954, when the Cooperative Research Act authorized "contracts or jointly financed cooperative arrangements with universities and colleges and state educational agencies for the conduct of research, surveys, and demonstrations in the field of education." With the National Defense Act of 1958, the Federal role in education was further increased to include administering large programs designed to improve schools, curricula, and teaching in order to encourage the development of talented youth. Then, with the Elementary and Secondary Education Act (ESEA) of 1965, the Government's role was further enlarged to designing programs to use in education as a means of attacking social problems such as discrimination and poverty. The Act further mandated that the new ESEA programs should be evaluated, thereby causing the government to need evaluation staff as well as program planners, analysts, and administrators. By 1970, the Government's role in education was very different from what it had been in 1954 and 1867.

Thus, the technical skills needed by the Government have shifted because of new tasks. They have also shifted because of new techniques. In this respect one need only think of the great strides made in all aspects of survey research methodology and how this has affected the Census Bureau—both in its census activities (e.g., how variables are measured, how interviewers comport themselves, how responses are processed) and its survey activities (how samples are drawn, how longitudinal data are analyzed, how surveys are costed).

The shift in technical skills can be seen by the kinds of people the government employs. At one time, lawyers were in great demand by Federal agencies because Government's role consisted largely of writing regulations and testing for compliance. Then, auditors came to play a major role, examining financial records. Next came economists, whose skills in projecting costs and estimating how expenditures in one area would affect another were in great demand. Lately, other kinds of social scientists have been in demand—those who know about needs assessment, program evaluation, and the measurement of social indicators. The Federal Government currently uses persons with all of these skills, but the skill mix changes from time to time.

The Comptroller General of the United States discusses these matters as follows (Statts, 1978):

Until about ten years ago, the GAO [General Accounting Office] staff was comprised almost entirely of accountants, who through training and development, became proficient in conducting management and program audits; in fact, most of GAO's top managers, who rose through the ranks, fall into that category.

In the mid-sixties, the United States Government became increasingly involved in solving social and environment problems and in procuring advanced weapon and space systems. The Congress wanted—and needed—to know whether these programs were working and whether they were worth the thousands of millions of Federal dollars invested in them. It soon became clear that, if GAO was to fulfill the role opening up to it, GAO would have to hire people with a wider range of skills and disciplines.*

The Politics of Federal Hiring

The increasing role of the government, its increasing need for technical skills, and the seemingly ever-changing nature of the skill mixes needed have to be seen in the context of two facts. One is that the size of the Federal Government is an important political issue. Politicians from both parties publicly pledge to cut back the size of Government, or at least reduce its growth, and many political groups regularly check on the total number of Federal employees and draw public attention to increases. Consequently, while Guttman & Willner (1976) estimated that the Federal budget increased from $70 billion to $500 billion over the past two decades, they estimated that the number of full-time civilian Federal employees had remained relatively stable.

The second important fact is that Federal employees at the professional level have job tenure after an initial probationary period. As a result, some persons hired at one time because of a particular skill continue to be employed even if their work is below the state of the art or irrelevant to needs at a later date. To be sure, the Federal Government institutes a wide variety of training programs to improve and modify the skill levels of its employees, but it is doubtful if training opportunities alone bring officials up to the state of the art level, except in rare instances.

A major reason why so many consulting services are needed today is that the demand for new technical skills has increased, while the supply of Federal officials cannot increase and the mix of their skills may be more appropriate to the needs of yesterday than today. Consulting services help fill the void between the amount and type of work asked of Government and the amount and type of work Government officials are able to perform themselves.

*From Statts, E.B. The General Accounting Office: Appraising science and technology programs in the United States. *Interdisciplinary Science Reviews*, 1978, *3*, 7–19.

Ideologic Factors

While the Federal Government relies heavily on contractors to provide goods and services needed to carry out its missions, a question arises as to what work must be done in-house and what may be contracted out. This problem of deciding whether the government should "make or buy" is reviewed in Chapter 6 of Part A of the Report of the U.S. Commission on Government Procurement (1972), which we will hereinafter refer to as the Commission Report. The Commission Report says that only limited expressions of policy in this regard appear in the statutes. Where policy is not determined by statute it must be inferred from executive branch policy statements and procedures. However, in the past these have been subject to controversy. OMB Circular A-76 (Policies for Acquiring Commercial or Industrial Products and Services for Government Use) states the policy currently in force. In general, criticality of need and relative cost to Government have been the primary factors in deciding the "make or buy" question.

There are differences, however, in the application of these criteria. Persons whom we might characterize as "conservative" believe that the private sector of our society is not being fostered as well as it should be and that the public sector is expanding too rapidly and is encroaching on the private sector. Conservatives are therefore particularly keen to prevent the number of federal employees from rising and so indirectly foster the use of consulting services. Actually, they sometimes foster it actively, as is made clear in a memorandum dated October 18, 1976 from James T. Lynn, Director of OMB under President Nixon. He writes that government policy reflects the fundamental concept that government should generally perform only those functions that are governmental in nature and should utilize the competitive incentives of the private enterprise system to provide the products and services necessary to support governmental functions. He therefore suggests "relying upon the private enterprise system to supply [Government's] need for . . . services, in preference to [Government] engaging in commercial or industrial activity" (e.g., conducting surveys or the like).

Populists also advocate more consultation, but less for the purpose of fostering contract research than to help Federal officials gain new perspectives on the problems they deal with. Of course, the perspective of concern to populists are those of the "general citizenry" or of the people directly affected by decisions rather than those of experts or interest groups. Many conservatives share the populist perspective on experts, and their call for boards being composed of persons affected by decisions may mean representatives of commerce and industry. In any event, both conservatives and populists call for a wider representation of outsiders in government and for a less intrusive role of government. Each of these expands the scope for consulting services.

Cost Concerns

One alternative to having contractors perform consulting services is to reduce the demands made on Government. This we do not consider likely. A second alternative is to have Government itself perform the services for which it currently pays consultants and contractors. This we also consider unlikely because of political pressures against expanding Government and political pressures to maintain the tenure system for Federal employees and because it might cost more for the Federal Government to perform services than it does to have the contract research industry perform them.

In the circular mentioned earlier, James Lynn specified to Federal agencies that they could perform services over and above their necessary Governmental services if and only if it cost the Government less to do the work itself than to contract with outsiders. Rarely will it cost the Government less, we feel, largely because Federal salaries tend to be higher than private industry salaries at all levels except the very top and because Federal benefits are higher. (In the circular Lynn specified that retirement benefits were considered to be 24.5 percent of base salary or wages!) Moreover, Federal overhead may be higher, although this is not at all clear. While no one knows if the work currently done by outside consultants could be performed at less expense by Federal employees, we doubt that it could. However, the issue is not pressing, and the need to resolve it would be acute only if the size of the present bureaucracy were to expand.

WHY IS THERE DISAFFECTION WITH CURRENT CONSULTING SERVICES?

The memorandum of President Carter and the inquiry of the Metcalf subcommittee express a tone of disaffection (at least in the sense of discomfort or disquiet) regarding Government's use of consulting services.

Disaffection about one aspect or another of Government activity is not uncommon and is frequently expressed by persons in and out of Government. It is not clear that disaffection is always warranted, particularly since the precise nature of the underlying issues and the causes of problems are often quite complex. Moreover, misplaced disaffection can sometimes lead to actions that have an adverse impact. We shall consider in some detail one recent example where the disaffection led to actions that increased costs without any associated improvement in quality.This example concerns the burden on the public of Government information collection and reporting requirements.

Government agencies collect a great deal of information from the public either directly by the agencies themselves or indirectly through contracts. Much of this information collection is mandated by law, such as employer reports of income tax withholdings of employees, although some of it is of the voluntary response type occurring as part of research. The research itself may be mandated by law (such as a major program evaluation), but individuals contacted as part of a research sample are rarely, if ever, compelled to fill out questionnaires as employers are about income tax withholdings. Government agencies collecting information from the public and Government contractors doing so in connection with work for a federal agency are required to have instruments reviewed and approved by OMB. Thus one way to reduce Federal reporting requirements is to reduce the number of approvals given by OMB, and in 1976 President Ford did exactly this. On March 1, 1976 he wrote to the Director of OMB saying

> American citizens are understandably exasperated by the complexity of reporting to the Federal Government....Specifically, I expect the number of reports which collect information from the public to be reduced by 10 percent by next June 30. Further, I expect you to undertake a continuing effort to reduce the burden of government reporting.

The impact of President Ford's instructions ultimately were felt disproportionately severely on the ''voluntary response'' category of information collection rather than the mandatory reporting category. This effect is discussed by Carter (1977) who reports on the cost increases generated by delays due to OMB form clearance without any associated improvement in the quality of the products.

Procedural Matters

The disaffection expressed in President Carter's memorandum concerns mostly procedural matters having to do with the appointment of consultants and contractors. One concern is with repeated appointments. The President's memorandum says this raises questions as to whether the work is better suited to other, more appropriate arrangements. The memorandum does not specify what these might be, but the President may have in mind that hiring the same person or firm year after year suggests that the skill in question ought to be learned by Government employees or that someone with the required skill should be permanently hired. If this is the case, there are problems with this argument in light of the difficulties of adding to the Federal bureaucracy and the time and effort it takes to learn a new technical skill. However, there may well be some instances where repeated appointments are not necessary, and a more vigorous scrutiny of repeat appointments might prove helpful. So, too, might a regulation mandating review procedures if a reappointment is to be made for longer than a specified period. The effectiveness of such a regulation would depend on who does the scrutiny, and whether the scrutiny would be of repeatedly used individuals and firms or whether it would be of tasks that are repeatedly performed externally, irrespective of who carried them out in the past. In any case, it seems to us that a scrutiny of repeated tasks might be more useful than a scrutiny of repeated appointments of individuals or firms.

President Carter's memorandum was also concerned with Federal agencies circumventing their staff ceilings by use of consultant arrangements. The consequence of this is to add to the staff without increasing the number of permanent employees. It is easy to see why agencies would want to do this, given their increased responsibilities and the political impossibility of expanding the regular staff. It is difficult to see what can be done to prevent this. A possible first step might be to impose more rigid limits on consulting and contracting, but this might have undesirable side effects analogous to those mentioned earlier resulting from reducing OMB clearance for information collection.

Another concern expressed in President Carter's memorandum was with conflicts of interest between consultants' advice and their other outside financial interests and affiliations; this arises most often when the vested interest is undisclosed. In fact, current practice does require disclosure by prospective consultants and contractors, so that in principle information should be available to reduce the occurrence of conflict situations.

The President's memorandum identifies another serious procedural concern: ". . . use of consultants to perform work of a policymaking or managerial nature which should be retained directly by agency officials." It is not always easy to establish how much contractors are encroaching on basic agency function, since there may be no clear indication of what these functions are. It has been alleged, however, that contractors have become what has been called the "Shadow Government," but this is not clear in the absence of an accepted definition of "essential Government functions."

Quality Concerns

Although procedural matters dominated President Carter's critique of consultants, the critique was not limited to such matters. He wrote about commissioned work not relevant in any obvious way to the agency's needs. There is a belief that this is more likely to happen toward the end of the fiscal year, when agencies obligate funds in order to show they are spending all their money. While it is not clear how the "end-of-the-year rush" contributes to the irrelevant contract phenomenon, page 157 of Volume III of the Commission Report (1972) suggests that it might in fact give rise to another problem: the use of grants rather than contracts because grants are quicker to process. The use or misuse of grants will be discussed more fully later. In any case, internal agency review procedures do call for critical analysis and justification of planned contracts so that in principle the irrelevant contract phenomenon can be controlled. This being the case, if there is indeed a problem of signifi-cant magnitude it would be advisable for critical analysis and justification of planned contracts to be carried out by persons outside the agency in question, which of course creates the dilemma of adding more consultants when efforts are being made to reduce their number.

Much of the disaffection with contractors that Federal officials and scholars raise stems from what is perceived to be the low technical quality of consulting work. One phenomenon affecting quality is best understood by contrasting the quality control that an organization can exercise over its own employees with the control that one organization (a Federal agency) can exercise over another (the contract firm). Within organizations, the emphasis is on evaluating employees in terms of the quality of their work, and regular performance ratings are made that involve tying individuals to specific tasks for which they take responsibility. As a result of these ratings—however pro forma—rewards ensue in the form of promotions, raises, and increased per-quisites. Also, informal rewards probably result, such as colleague respect and increased influence. There is usually also a formal system of negative actions including warnings, reprimands, suspension, firing, and closing or reorganizing whole organizational units; informal aspects of negative action include decreased influence and responsibility, reduced quality of working conditions, and low colleague opinion.

In practice it is not easy to implement the kind of quality control system for in-house employees that we have just described because of tenure, senior-ity, and fixed salary features, which often reduce what a supervisor can do. Moreover, costly appeal procedures make it difficult to apply negative sanc-tions. Nonetheless, if it is difficult for an organization to maintain quality control internally, consider the restricted control possibilities that an agency has with respect to external contractors. A person working on a contract is evaluated as an employee of the contracting organization rather than of the agency paying for the contract. While the contracting organization has a stake in the quality of the work, the contractor's agenda and priorities are different from those of the sponsoring agencies, for the contractor, getting the contract is at least as important as doing the work. Consequently, a contractor's inter-ests imperfectly represent the interests of the sponsoring government agency, and the employees of a contract research firm will be evaluated in terms of the contractor's criteria of success and not in terms of the agency's criteria of quality work. However, the Government does have mechanisms for control-ling the quality of work of contractors. These include withholding of payment for work done that is not up to the quality desired and the potential to stop work on a contract or cancel it. These sanctions are powerful and are probably more easily applied in cases of gross malfeasance than in marginal cases of perceived low quality.

A number of mechanisms exist in contract research firms to promote quality work. Within the firm, contracts of moderate and large size may be worked on by several professionals and other staff members so that, while responsibility is formally on the principal investigator's shoulders, a large part of the planning and execution would involve team rather than individual efforts. Also, drafts of reports can be read and discussed by in-house colleagues, although the prevalence of this varies considerably from firm to firm. Liberal use is also made of outside technical consultants whose expenses are charged to the contract and who help develop or critique questionnaires or data analysis plans. Use is also made of advisory boards, which, with larger contracts, are frequently mandated. Quality is also enhanced, of course, by professional pride and the desire to maintain a good reputation, both individually and corporately. The strength of these mechanisms varies from one firm to another and from one individual to another.

Some firms take corporate responsibility for their work. They may, as was mentioned earlier, designate a senior management official as responsible for each contract and provide for technical quality and management review before a completed report can go to a contracting agency. However, there is disagreement about the value of review. John McGee, president of Arthur D. Little, Inc., is quoted in the *Wall Street Journal* of May 27, 1977 as saying that "we don't want the review process to have a dominance (that would) weaken the responsibility of the case leader; a review process can't build quality." In any case, many firms do not take organizational responsibility for the quality of their products, and responsibility rests with the principal investigator employed by the firm. Since low-quality work is the investigator's fault and not the firm's, there is not the same incentive to review documents.*

Sponsoring agencies must frequently take the blame for poor quality. The Committee on Fundamental Research Relevant to Education (National Research Council, 1977) states in its final report (p. 64), "Even more serious are those projects that contradict what is known scientifically, build on an inadequate base of knowledge, are ill-designed to fill gaps in understanding, or require quick, predictable answers from science that are inherently impos-

---

*Concerns about consulting are also voiced by individuals who work for the more famous, larger contracting firms.Their concern is directed at the many small consulting firms, some of which are set up just to bid on a particular contract and then disappear or reemerge for another RFP with a different name and some changes in personnel. Others are established by former government employees or by academics who seek to augment their salaries (a contract with their university would not allow payment over and above regular salary) or to bypass what are considered to be excessive bureaucratic requirements. Many individuals within the larger contracting organizations believe that the smaller, fly-by-night operations give the contracting business a bad name. This belief cannot be tested easily, but it has some credibility in that the larger, established organizations are vulnerable in the long term if they begin to be associated with inferior work performed by smaller companies.

sible to achieve.'' The Committee goes on to cite specific examples of badly drawn RFPs that embody these quality problems.

The quality of research can also be adversely affected by bad agency monitoring. Contractors frequently perceive agency monitors as arbitrary and capricious, asking for frequent changes in the nature and direction of the work. Moreover, if there is an agency change in the monitor during the course of a contract, the contractor may have to expend considerable effort in establishing a satisfactory working relationship with the new monitor, which may involve substantive changes in the work. A contractor might also be caught in a web of agency politics that results in shifting the scope of work while the project is in progress. All of these things make it difficult to maintain a focus on the quality of the work.

Low quality of work must also be interpreted in light of the severe budget and time constraints affecting contracted research. Because cost is a factor in the awarding of a contract, the system discourages contractors from asking for and agency monitors from recommending cost increases to improve quality without an evident increase in the scope of work. Similarly, Federal agencies are so often under pressure to produce results that they find it difficult to approve even reasonable time extensions for projects in the interest of improving quality.

Finally, it must be noted that there is considerable heterogeneity among both agency personnel and contractors. Some are better than others. Thus it is difficult to generalize about quality and unfair to ascribe deficiencies in specific terms. Moreover, many of the arguments we have presented very likely can cut both ways. The very nature of the relationship between Government agency and contractor presents potential for problems. On one hand the agency must exercise control if the work is to address its missions, while on the other hand sufficient latitude must be given the performer for creative work. As Young (1978) puts it, ''Thus a delicate balance requiring a high degree of judgement must be struck in the relationships between executive agencies and performing institutions in the procurement of R & D [Research and Development].''

SUGGESTIONS FOR IMPROVEMENT

An obstacle to any rational discussion of consulting services is the absence of valid data about the volume and cost of such services in the various agencies comprising the Federal Government. The publication by OMB of proposed ''Guidelines for Use of Consultant Services'' (Federal Register, Vol. 42, December 17, 1977, pp. 63492−63493) is a step toward improving the current situation, since the Guidelines explicitly address issues about monitoring the number and cost of contractors. Indeed, the Federal Procurement Data System (FPDS) referred to by OMB is now operational, and the report should be publicly available by April, 1979. Although the Metcalf subcommittee raised questions as to whether or not the FPDS will deal adequately with all of the data problems, it seems clear that a start has been made.

The OMB Guidelines deal with *basic* policy as well as data requirements. The following important policy points are made:

1. Consultant services will not be used to make policy or management decisions, since these will be retained directly by agency officials.
2. Consultant services will be obtained only on an intermittent or temporary basis; repeated or extended arrangements are not to be entered into.
3. Consultant services will not be used as a device to bypass or undermine personnel ceiling, pay limitations, or competitive employment procedures.
4. Former Government employees will not be given preference in consultant service arrangements.

Elsewhere the proposed OMB Guidelines state that each agency will assure for all consultant service arrangements that

1. Every requirement for consultant services is appropriate and fully justified in writing, and such justification will also certify that a complete search of available agency studies, reports, or similar information has been conducted, that such information differs from current requirements, and what new information is to be collected;
2. Work statements for consultant services are specific, complete, and specify a fixed period of performance for the service to be provided;
3. In the case of contracts for consultant services, contracts are competitively awarded to the maximum extent to ensure that costs are reasonable;
4. Appropriate disclosure and warning provisions are given to the performer(s) to avoid conflict of interest;
5. Consultant service arrangements are properly administered and monitored to ensure that performance is satisfactory.

These "policies" and "management controls" address most of the procedural concerns expressed in President Carter's memorandum, and they can be applied to individual consultation, advisory board consultation, and individual contract firms. The major issue is how the provisions will be implemented in practice and whether or not the payoff from their implementation will be greater than the financial and administrative costs of following the proposed Guidelines.

Comprehensive Changes

A full understanding of Government procurement of research through contracts requires examination of the broader context of roles and responsibilities that occur in various transactions and relationships between the Federal Government and non-Federal parties. An extensive and thoughtful review of these relationships has recently been completed (Young, 1978) and what follows in the next four paragraphs stems from Young's work.

The Federal procurement system (as regulated by the Federal Procurement Regulations) is designed for the purchase of goods and services for the direct benefit or use of the Federal Government. The legal instrument reflecting the relationship is the contract. The primary responsibility for the work is the Government's; the Government involvement during performance varies but can be whatever is necessary to be consistent with the Federal Procurement Regulations. Also, the Government usually has the unilateral right to redirect the work or terminate it. When procurement of hardware was the dominant use of contracts, the sealed-bid fixed-price approach was the typical mode. Following the Second World War, as the Government contracted for more and more research greater flexibility was introduced (e.g., negotiated contracts) in recognition of the special problems occurring, such as when an agency's needs cannot be fully specified at the outset. As Young says, "The adaptation of the procurement system to mobilize the nation's scientific and technical talents has produced a whole series of remarkable technological accomplishments in the military and space areas." The effectiveness of contracting in this regard was possible because the Government was indeed the user of the results.

Now, however, the Government is more and more active in the support of R & D to meet civil sector needs in energy, environment, health, housing, transportation, education, training, and law enforcement. Unlike military and space departments, the users of the knowledge generated in these areas are not only the Federal Government but also private individuals and companies as well as state and local governments. This raises the question as to whether the same procurement system can be simply redirected toward meeting civil sector needs or whether more fundamental changes are required.

In recognition of these and other problems, the Federal Grant and Cooperative Agreement Act of 1977 (P.L. 95-224) was enacted, establishing a framework to clarify the roles and responsibilities that occur when non-Federal parties become involved with the Federal Government through procurement of assistance. This Act requires that assistance relationships be distinguished as a class from procurement relationships and establishes criteria for the use of contracts, grants, and cooperative agreements so that these legal instruments reflect the underlying relationships between Government agencies and non-Federal parties. *Procurement contracts* are to be used (as described above) to purchase goods or services for use by the Government. The Government has significant authority and responsibility and may be substantially involved in performance. *Assistance* refers to transfer of funds to accomplish a public purpose of support or stimulation authorized by Federal statute rather than acquisition or purchase. Within the assistance category, *grants* are used when responsibility for performance is delegated to the recipient, and there is to be little or no Federal involvement in performance. *Cooperative agreements* are to be used in cases of shared Government–recipient responsibility for performance and where there is to be substantial Government involvement during performance.

Recognizing that it is only a first step, the Federal Grant and Cooperative Agreement Act mandates a two-year comprehensive study of Federal assistance to be conducted by the Director of the OMB. It seems to us that the reexamination now going on of the precise nature of the various transactions and relationships that occur between the Government and non-Federal parties may hold promise for clarifying roles and responsibilities and may lead to higher-quality contracted research. Moreover, we believe that the concept of shared responsibility associated with cooperative agreements holds promise for improving the quality and utility of civil sector R & D that might formerly have been done by contract.

We now turn to what we believe would be another important change that can be taken at the comprehensive level of Government: inclusion of information about a contractor's past performance in the Government's data system on consulting and contracting. This information could then be used in contractor selection.

Using past performance information raises many practical difficulties, including the possibility of being unfair to contractors when judgmental information is included in the record. However, some kinds of information are not judgmental and will not be so controversial. For instance, the data system might include information about the actual completion date and the final cost of each contract, perhaps with agency comments about why a proposed completion date was not met or why there were cost overruns. It is certainly important to know whether delays and increases in costs came about because of difficulties in, say, getting OMB clearances for data collection instruments, or from agency changes in the scope of work, or from poor estimates by the contractor.

The program office of the sponsoring agency must currently certify to the agency's business or contracting office that the contract work was completed and of acceptable quality. These certifications have no "teeth" at present, largely because requests for payment are treated routinely and may not be directly associated with substantive performance, but this situation could easily be changed, perhaps by withholding 10 percent of the total contract costs until an acceptable final report is delivered. The rules governing this would have to be very carefully worked out; withholding payment opens the door to potentially abusive treatment of contractors by agencies. Certifications would be more useful for accountability purposes if they were detailed enough to be used in making future awards, but since a more detailed certification would inevitably entail judgments on the part of the agency, contractors ought to have an opportunity for rebuttal. A contractor's final report could also be sent out for external review, with the results also becoming part of the system for procurement decisions. If reviews are used for this purpose, great care is needed in deciding which persons should do the reviewing, by what standards they should make judgments, and in which format they should respond.

In fact, past performance is usually taken into account in selection, and sometimes persons are named to selection panels precisely because of their knowledge of the past performance of bidding organizations. However, such information is not used systematically, and there are few guidelines for its use. Moreover, the techniques we have mentioned (e.g., reviews of final reports) are also used in some cases and by some offices within agencies; however, they are not used systematically or in a way that would allow the Government to improve on the techniques through aggregation of experience across agencies.

Agency Level Changes

Sometimes grants are used to support projects that should be done by contract. We mentioned that this seems to occur more often during the end-of-the-year rush because grants are easier to process than contracts. It also may be natural for an agency program manager to prefer grants to contracts because grants reduce his monitoring responsibilities. However, it has been our experience that there is sometimes a tendency for ideologic reasons to prefer grants to contracts in support of research. This point of view holds that creativity is fostered by allowing those actually doing the research as much freedom and flexibility as possible, which is the norm in a grant situation. Furthermore, agency interest in the work can be represented informally through contacts between grantees and agency personnel.

But treating grants like contracts is problematic. First, since informal understandings about grants have no enforceability, misunderstandings and disagreements may occur without there being any formal procedures for resolving them. Second, an undesirable coercive climate may develop. Researchers may resent what agency people want to do with a grant but endure it in silence out of fear of agency retaliation at the next grant funding cycle. Third, government procurement through grants is one of the abuses the Presideht and the Congress are trying to correct. Grants are intended to support what the scholars in a particular substantive area want to do, not what the Government wants done. In fact, this is one of the problems that the Federal Grant and Cooperative Agreement Act addresses. As experience is gained under this Act, one would hope that misuse of grants will decrease.

It is crucial for an agency to decide on the purpose of a piece of research, which in turn will determine the degree of Government control required and whether the assistance or procurement mode of funding is appropriate. Then the appropriate instrument (grant, cooperative agreement, or contract) can be used. The quality of contract research would be facilitated considerably if Federal officials gave more thought to what should be a contract rather than a grant and if, in particular instances, they discussed with their colleagues what they hoped to gain from a particular contract.

Once an information need has been identified that a contract might meet, the next step is to advertise or to contact a prospective performer. Frequently, this step involves issuance of an RFP. Here, as the OMB Guidelines suggest, it is important for work statements to be specific and comprehensive, particularly with respect to the period of performance, level of effort, and outputs expected. To be sure, the bidder must be able to exercise some creative ingenuity in the design and methodology of the research, but the agency must be clear about purposes, audiences, scope, etc. Otherwise, bidders will have trouble writing proposals, and proposal evaluation will be complicated and perhaps even unfair.

As earlier described, the selection of a contractor depends on the quality of the proposal, the cost of the research, and the contractor's presumed capability to carry out the work. Since most of the review of submitted proposals is carried out within an agency, the selection panel can often neglect important technical details that might vitiate good research. Also, it is not clear that the agency personnel can represent the interests of the various constituencies with a stake in the research results. Further, the absence of information about the *representative* work done by a particular firm or principal investigator in the past makes it difficult to check on the track record of the persons proposing to do the research. This problem is exacerbated because the people who will actually work on the project are not always the same persons who are listed in the proposal. Although the agency can do something about this, it may not always be aware that it is happening. In any case, the cardinal rule is that proposals stand by themselves. In this respect is is important to note that the way a proposal is written can significantly help chances of being funded, and sometimes organizations that could best perform the work are eliminated because of poorly written proposals. Thus the art of proposal writing is extremely important, and the best resources of organizations are devoted to this. Consequently, proposal review requires considerable skill, judgement, and insight.

We strongly suspect that the review of contract proposals can be improved by (1) bringing the views of outside experts to bear, (2) checking on past research records more thoroughly, and (3) extracting guarantees that the people listed in the proposal will actually work on the project so long as they remain in the employ of the firm in question. Some agencies have made considerable effort to build rating schemes for evaluating proposals and to assay reliability of the ratings. Such efforts are commendable and should be disseminated among agencies.

One of the most difficult aspects of quality control is the oversight and "technical direction" that occurs from the moment the contract is let and lasts until the final report is accepted. We refer to all this as *monitoring*. Monitoring is concerned with such matters as (1) whether or not the work is progressing on schedule and with the agreed rate of expenditures of funds, (2) whether or not the agreed-upon personnel—especially key personnel—are working on the project in the expected capacity and with the agreed level of effort, (3) whether or not the key project personnel perceive any problems with which the monitor might be able to help, (4) whether or not any changes in the proposed project are occuring and, if so, why, and (5) whether or not the major substantive performance milestones are being met.

A particularly difficult monitoring issue is the detection of problems early to correct them, which sometimes requires site visits and the maintenance of informed telephone contact with the project. However, interim reports are usually more useful to the monitor and probably can be made less burdensome to all if they are scheduled to coincide with substantive performance milestones rather than an arbitrary chronology. For example, instrument development is vital to most social science studies, and if it is to be completed in month 4 of a contract, it is more important to get a report at that time than to receive some arbitrarily scheduled quarterly report in month 3. Interim reports should be substantive rather than descriptive; thus they should include copies of the instruments for agency review and approval rather than just stating that instrument development is complete. Substantive reports at crucial project milestones need not add to the reporting burden, since they will usually be drafts of chapters that will appear in the final report. Indeed, keeping a clear focus on the final report helps both monitors and contractors, and all intervening activities can be seen as preliminary attempts at revising and fleshing out the final report.

At various steps along the way, the agency will need to review and approve such technical aspects of a contracted project as sampling plans, instruments, data analysis plans, and so forth. The single individual who is the agency monitor may not embody all the skills and expertise required for adequate review of all these matters. Thus the monitor and the monitor's superiors ought to be open to occasionally organizing small heterogeneous teams of monitors; they should be prepared to call in external consultants with the requisite expertise when necessary. For long, complex projects, continuity in monitoring is essential; thus small teams of monitors and perhaps consultants should be signed up for the duration of a contract. [A discussion of this use of consultants, including the need for continuity, is given by Cook & Gruder (1978) under the heading of Consultant Metaevaluation.]

Two project milestones seem to us to be particularly important. The first is the first interim report, which gives a first check on the quality of the contract work, indicates special problems that have arisen in implementing a planned research design in the field, and permits the project director and agency monitor to interact for the first time on a substantive matter. The degree to which they are comfortable working together, monitor reassurance about quality and project director reassurance that the agency is not unnecessarily intrusive are important indicators of how smooth the course is likely to be over the life of the project. More important is the fact that the first interim report provides the earliest information *from the field* about how the contract is progressing and what modifications—if any—need to be made in order to gain the contract's objectives now that field relationships and feasibility constraints are clearer. We would like to see more thought devoted to first interim reports with respect to linking them to the most crucial initial mileposts of a contract, making them more comprehensive than they currently are, using them for the explicit purpose of bringing up implementation problems at an early date and trying to solve these problems before it is too late.

When the first draft of the final report arrives, the agency will usually want to give it a rigorous reading, including a reading by outsiders. Comments provided by reviewers are given to the project director, who is expected to incorporate them into revisions. This is a delicate time. Although the need for revision is acknowledged, the mood of a project group when it submit that first draft of the final report is that the work is virtually over. Indeed, by that time many of the project staff will have been assigned to new projects tht pay their salaries. Although the remaining staff usually want to repair major errors, they may resist extensive revisions, particularly if funds are low and there is a problem in paying for the revisions. This is probably why the completion of a final report often requires cost overruns and extensions in the period of contract performance. Since decisions about extensions of time and money have to be justified by the monitor's superiors, and since the monitor may fear that asking for extensions will reflect badly on him, pressures exist to accept a final report of inferior quality. Our earlier suggestions to keep the final report clearly in mind from the outset and to devise interim reports to foreshadow it will be helpful in preparing higher-quality drafts. The agency monitor therefore ought to work out his review plan and schedule well in advance and process the drafts expeditiously.

The second difficult monitoring issue involves delineating the limits of the monitor's role and the contractor's responsibilities. This difficulty arises most often when monitors and hired consultants suggest changes to contractors that they do not want to make but feel they must. But it also arises because many projects, especially large and complicated ones, have their own advisory boards and consultants who are supposed to help the project director. These persons are also potentially helpful to the agency monitor, who may wish to ensure that the agency has approval rights concerning all consultants and advisors and that all consultant and advisory board reports go directly to the agency monitor as well as the project director. Treating consultants who are paid from contracts in this way is a delicate matter; it is not clear whether the consultants work for the sponsoring agency or the project. We recommend against agency heavyhandedness in these matters, but the contractors should recognize that an agency's willingness to pay the cost of advisory boards and consultants is directly related to the need to examine substantive work by the advisors and consultants.

Another aspect of this problem arises in terms of the balance of responsibility for creative initiative between contractor and agency. In procurement contracting, the agency is ultimately responsible for assuring performance, which is a key distinction from assistance grants. In the latter case, the agency discharges its responsibility through monitoring intended to fulfill purposes of accountability and quality control. The contractor is expected to do the work. If a contract involves, say, development of a questionnaire, it is usually the contractor's responsibility to submit to the agency a questionnaire that is the result of significant substantive effort and that is close to a final version. The contractor should not expect the agency monitor, in clarifying the broad requirements of the RFP, to provide substantive assistance in questionnaire design (except, of course, in the exceptional situation where the contract makes such a provision). Unfortunately, creativity on the part of the contractor may not always be appreciated and can lead to extra work, especially if it is seen as departing from the specifications in the contract. Moreover, agency monitors have been known to request frequent redirections of the work that can inhibit creativity and even lower quality.

Monitoring is a duty of public employees, not a power that they usurp. Consequently, agency monitors and contractors would do well to work together as professional colleagues in an atmosphere of trust. With this in mind, we suggest the following guidelines for monitoring: First, major substantive advice, guidance, recommendations, etc. from the monitor should be in writing in order to minimize misunderstandings. Second, it is the contractor's responsibility to determine what is to be done about the advice, guidance, recommendations, etc. (when these are not directives). Third, in the understanding that the monitor's "advice," even when not a "directive," can cause substantive change, the written record should provide a basis for public and professional accountability. Finally, if really significant differences between the contractor and the agency occur that do not involve charges of nonperformance, then mutually acceptable adjudication by third parties should be arranged.

CONCLUSIONS

We see a clear trend suggesting a future expansion of the Federal Government's role with respect to monitoring the condition of the nation. This trend will mean an increase in the amount and nature of information collected from Americans. We also foresee the possibility that the Government may be even more involved in service delivery programs. Although the role of Government may increase in either or both of these respects, it is unlikely that there will be corresponding increases in the number of people working for the Federal Government, which means that the Government will have to contract for social research and that the Government's use of consulting services will have to increase in the future. For a variety of reasons, the increase is more likely to occur with contract research firms rather than with individual consultants or advisory boards.

We also expect that disaffection with the Government's use of consulting services will flare up from time to time because of such inherent conflicts as a call for more input from the constituencies affected by Government as contrasted with the call to reduce consultation overall; the call to use less expensive services outside of a Federal agency versus the call not to farm out agency functions; or the call to have contract work performed versus the call to appear "efficient" by not funding proposal writing or professionals who are between contracts.

Both the President and Congress have made progress in identifying many of the concerns about consulting services and in producing guidelines for improvement. However, these efforts give considerable emphasis to such front-end concerns as contractor selection and, in our opinion, not enough emphasis to issues affecting the relevance and quality of the final outputs. Our principal recommendations for improving quality include increasing the rewards and sanctions that can be brought to bear for high- or poor-quality work and improving the sophistication of monitoring so that problems can be detected early enough to be corrected.

REFERENCES

Carter, J. E., Memorandum from the President to heads of executive departments and agencies, May 12, 1977.

Carter, L. F. Federal clearance of education instruments: Procedural problems and proposed remedies. *Educational Researcher,* 1977, *6,* 7−12.

Cater, D., & Strickland, L. *TV violence and the child.* New York: Russell Sage Foundation, 1975.

Cook, T. D., & Gruder, C. L. Meta-evaluation research. *Evaluation Quarterly,* 1978, *2,* 5−51.

Guttman, D., & Willner, B. *The shadow government.* New York: Pantheon Books, 1976.

Kelling, G. L. *Development of staff for evaluations (a retrospective view), emergency medical services: Research methodology* (DHEW Publication No. 78-3195). Washington, D.C.: U.S. GPO, 1977.

National Research Council, Committee on Fundamental Research Relevant to Education. *Fundamental research and the process of education.* Washington, D.C.: National Academy of Sciences, 1977.

Office of Management and Budget. Proposed guidelines for use of consultant services. *Federal Register,* 1977, *42,* 63492−63493.

Office of Management and Budget. Policies for acquiring commercial or industrial products and services for Government use. OMB Transmittal Memorandum No. 2. *Federal Register,* 1976, *41,* 46528.

Statts, E. B. The General Accounting Office: Appraising science and technology programs in the United States. *Interdisciplinary Science Reviews,* 1978, *3,* 7−19.

Subcommittee on Reports, Accounting and Management of the Committee on Governmental Affairs of the United States Senate. Consultants and Contractors, A Survey of the Government's Purchase of Outside Services. Washington, D.C.: U.S. GPO, 1977.

U.S. Commission on Government Procurement. *Report of the Commission on Government Procurement,* (5 vols.). Washington, D.C.: U.S. GPO, 1972.

Young, J. H. Applications of R & D in the civil sector: The opportunity provided by the Federal Grant and Cooperative Agreement Act of 1977. Report of the Office of Technology Assessment of the U.S. Congress, 1978.

C. Abraham Fenster,
Harvey Schlossberg

6

The Psychologist as Police
Department Consultant

There are no explicit legal requirements for becoming a police department
psychologist. We consider the psychologist's personal maturity and emotional
stability, including the ability to withstand stress and personal flexibility, as
crucial as the technical knowledge brought to the scene. Psychologists who
work with or for police will often come under attack from their professional
("liberal"?) colleagues, since, unfortunately, psychologists share many negative beliefs about police (Reiser, 1970). At psychological meetings, police
department psychologists are not only asked to defend their own performance
but are also called upon to defend police brutality, traffic citations, prejudicial
attitudes, and departmental police operations. Especially in the 1960s, so-
called liberal and radical social scientists came to see police as the enemy and
tended to stereotype anyone who worked with or for the police department as
"one of them." As psychologists who have worked with and taught police
officers, we emphatically reject this point of view. The psychologist who is a
police department consultant is realistically working for change instead of just
talking about it, recognizing the need for change but striving to achieve such
change cooperatively and realistically. Psychologists acting as police consultants must have the strength of their convictions, must anticipate attack and
not be overly sensitive to such onslaught, and should be able to defend their
positions without being either overly abrasive or apologetic. Because there is
always resistance to change and especially to agents of such change, much
patience and some tolerance for frustration is required (Reiser, 1971).

Consulting psychologists must be especially careful not to stereotype
policemen and must continually examine their own biases, whether positive or
negative. Psychologists must examine their own unresolved power needs as

well as their own unresolved conflicts in relation to authority figures. Just as psychotherapists must be aware of their own irrational biases toward their patients (countertransferences), if they are to be effective in dealing with their patients, so too must psychologists consulting to police departments.

Police department psychologists must be realistic in their expectations. They must realize that in bureaucratic hierarchic organizations "evolution rather than revolution is the mode of change" (Reiser, 1972). They will encounter strong vested interests, many power struggles, and much resistance to change.

Despite some suggestions and some limited opportunities for interdisciplinary graduate training in forensic psychology (Brodsky, 1976; Fenster, Litwack, & Symonds, 1975; 1976; Fenster, 1976), most police department consultants will have their doctoral degrees in clinical and other traditional areas of psychology. Police department consulting psychologists should be skilled in research design and evaluation, individual and group psychotherapy, industrial psychology, and community relations. Above all, they must be flexible enough to take on the widest range of requests for services and not set rigid, *a priori* limits on their roles. It is essential, however, that they keep in mind that they are employed by the organization and have specific roles and responsibilities within the organization's structure. They must be on guard not to attempt change or manipulate in conformity with their own needs rather than those for whom they are responsible.

In dealing with hostage situations—a "new" kind of crisis—the need for flexibility on the part of both police psychologists and police officers themselves can be illustrated. Police are trained to be people of action; the public expects this of them. In hostage situations, however, no action is often the best action (Schlossberg & Freeman, 1974); since boredom, the desire to escape, and hunger all become paramount needs over time and since a male perpetrator feels less of a threat to his masculinity over time, the hostages will virtually always be saved. Police psychologists can often teach police officers to reexamine some of the techniques that they have by trial and error experience come to use. They can help officers organize their experiences and give insight as to which techniques can best be used in various crisis situations. The psychologist's role, then becomes one of combining academic knowledge with practical expertise. Psychologist consultants, then, in their involvement find that they are working *with* the police, not *for* them, by enabling working police officers to reach their potentials.

RELATIONSHIP OF THE CONSULTING PSYCHOLOGIST TO THE POLICE DEPARTMENT

Consulting psychologists must be familiar with police work. Typically, they should observe (and maybe even participate in) the recruit training program, read the training manual and other literature put out by the department, and visit special divisions such as jail, narcotics, internal affairs, vice, etc. Psychologists should read the literature, ride in patrol cars, and talk with patrol officers, supervisors, administrators, and police department instructors at every opportunity so as to continually "marinate" in police department matters.

In working with police departments, psychologists must strive to make themselves known in the department and be accepted as nonthreatening experts. Psychologists should not be unduly formal or forbidding.

Police department psychologists are often involved in obtaining research grants, modifying police department procedures, publishing research, writing articles for magazines and scholarly journals, lecturing at colleges and universities, giving talks at schools, churches, or business meetings, or being interviewed on radio and television. Some of these activities receive various degrees of notice by the public.

Police have ambivalent reactions to consulting psychologists. While police may be dazzled by the psychologist's ease with words and by the title "doctor" and may ascribe omnipotence to the psychologist, they will also feel threatened by the psychologist's potential for danger as a "mind reader." Consequently, the consulting psychologist must be aware of resistance from all levels of the police department.

It is crucial that psychologist-consultants to the police department work with a top-level administrator on a day-to-day basis if their suggestions are to be meaningfully evaluated and adopted. Psychologists should exert influence through the entire department structure. If they get connected only to the lower levels of the department, there is a strong risk that nobody will pay attention to them and that their recommendations will not get very far. There should not be much distance between the consultants and the managers of an organization (Levinson, 1970), since consultants' roles are largely dependent on the functions they are expected to perform (Gilbert, 1960). Consultants need sufficient status and power so that many of their suggestions get implemented and so that their identification and commitment to the department get strengthened (Reiser, 1972). Because police administrators may unconsciously fear "magical powers" of psychologist-consultants, police psychologists must have the personal adaptability to come across as nonthreatening, rational, pragmatic, and helpful.

While psychologists should work with the upper echelons of the police department, they should have access to decision makers and managers at all levels by attending meetings, holding conferences, and writing in police department magazines or training bulletins (Burger, 1970). They should maintain liaison with other professional groups, presenting papers and attending professional meetings. Consultants must accept the general organizational goals if their work is to be successful. If consultants have great needs for respect and status and feel that their image of themselves as experts must be maintained at all costs and are therefore reluctant to communicate their knowledge, they will fail (Hodges, 1970).

Consulting psychologists need to remember that their expertise lies in the direction of providing information, suggesting new options, and evaluating police practices and their implications. Competing individuals and "pressure groups" will attempt to get them to make "professional" decisions that are really beyond their responsibility. Here psychologists must be firm, although gentle, in setting limits. Otherwise, they could well get involved in organizational conflicts that will erode their usefulness to the organization. Here psychologists must be aware of their own grandiose needs and power drives, which may sabotage their effectiveness.

PROVIDING DIRECT SERVICES

Counseling, Psychotherapy, and Police Personality

Consulting psychologists often supervise or directly provide psychotherapy and counseling services to police personnel and their families. Here marital problems are most common, although the complete spectrum of psychotherapy problems handled by the private practitioner may appear. Psychologists have obligations to clearly spell out the limits of their confidentiality. When police officers seek psychotherapy voluntarily, confidentiality should be maintained; otherwise police officers will avoid psychologists rather than seeking them out. In rare and unusual circumstances when after entering into a confidential relationship with a police psychologist an officer becomes psychotic, seriously criminal, or suicidal or begins acting-out in a very destructive fashion, the need for confidentiality is overridden by the paramount consideration of protecting the patient and the community. However, any violations of confidentiality are very serious. Infringements of confidentiality must be kept to a minimum. When a police officer is referred for counseling, psychotherapy, psychodiagnosis, or evaluation, the psychologist obligated to report back to the referral sources must so inform the officer client at the outset (Schlossberg & Freeman, 1974).

Often therapy will have to be brief, using some of the more active approaches and ideas, or outside referrals will have to be made. For example, group therapy sessions have become excellent means of both training police officers in new techniques and helping them deal with anxieties and inadequacies. Psychologists help form various groups and determine their goals. They can act as either facilitators or therapists, and they can help the officers understand the goals of the organization or help them understand their own aggressive impulses.

Many dedicated officers at some point in their careers encounter difficulties not considered to be of psychiatric proportions; however, because of the stress of police work assistance may be needed. Consultants earn their salaries in these situations by eliminating many of the problems before they are carried into the field. The triple benefit obviously is increased productivity for the organization, increased performance for the community, and a more fulfilled individual.

Another example of short-term therapy use involves marriage counseling. Realizing that many of the problems faced at home are the result of displaced anxiety, stress, and aggression that would be further displaced to the public, we can block the process by providing therapy. We recognize that the police department is not in the treatment business, but prevention of disorders that could adversely affect performance is both economically and morally a responsibility. In line with these demands, consultants must use innovative methods; for example, videotape therapy for marital problems is opening new frontiers in short-term treatment.

Often consulting psychologists are asked to evaluate employees in terms of emotional status, ability to carry a gun, etc. Sometimes they are asked for formal diagnostic evaluations using personality tests as well. It is fair to say that the value of a formal diagnosis in and of itself is questionable and that diagnoses have often been abused. Consulting psychologists should be familiar with mental health referral sources in the community as well as resources for dealing with problems involving legal aid, pregnancy, abortion, child welfare services, school, and employment placement. However, the needs of the individual are paramount. Consulting psychologists must be aware of and sensitive to situations that could lead to the abuse of their offices. Particularly in a bureaucratic organization, it is the responsibility of psychologists to make sure that their services are not used as punitive measures or as substitute for administrative or supervisory procedures. However, this does not mean that they disregard responsibilities to the police department in such cases where disorder is adverse to the functioning of the department, i.e., types of psychopathic or malingering behavior.

To function effectively police officers need to feel secure and worthwhile and have positive self-images. Free counseling and psychotherapy should be available to police officers who request it, since many would benefit greatly (Runkel, 1971; Brodsky, 1976). While officers may seek or be referred for psychotherapy for the same problems that affect other people, e.g., marital difficulties, psychosomatic disturbances, excessive drinking, sexual acting-out, neurosis, character disturbances, or traumatic situational personality disorders, there is evidence of different types of occupational personalities (Walther, 1964).

Sociologists tend to account for this difference by speaking of the effects of occupational and institutional pressures influencing and shaping the individual. Accordingly, Niederhoffer (1967) speaks of the special type of authoritarian personality required by the police role, the system shaping the mind of police officers so that they feel righteous and justified when they use power and toughness in carrying out duties. Similarly, Skolnick (1966) feels that since police officers must habitually attend to potentially dangerous or violent situations, good police officers become "suspicious" individuals who then grow mistrustful and isolated from the citizens whom they now "suspect" as sources of danger. When this feeling gets generalized onto the larger community, a situation arises of social distance between police officers and most segments of the community. This kind of induced "paranoia" as a personality trait has some parallels to etiology of the "suspiciousness" prevalent among minority groups (Grier & Cobbs, 1968). Similar sociologic views are presented by others (Astor, 1971; Bayler & Mendelsohn, 1969; Brown, 1971; Dodd, 1967; Murphy, 1965; Radano, 1968; Westley, 1953; Whelton, 1971).

In contrast to the sociologic viewpoint that the job shapes the worker, psychologists generally believe that different or special types of people are drawn to police work as a kind of sublimation (Rapaport, 1949) and that personality needs play an important part in the choice of a career (Roe, 1956). Thus recruit screening becomes one of the prime considerations for police consultants. They must devise innovative methods in the use of existing screening procedures as well as devise research aimed at defining the needs of police work. The qualities of trait clusters that would make for success in police work have proved elusive to researchers (Schlossberg, 1974).

Much of the research and scholarly writing is contradictory concerning the nature of police personality. For example, police officers were either found to be or thought of as mentally unstable (New York Times, 1964; Rankin, 1959), schizoid (Rapaport, 1949), secretive (Clark, 1965; Glazer, 1958; Stoddard, 1968; Westley, 1951; 1956), suspicious (Glaser, 1958; Matarazzo, Allen, Saslow, & Wiens, 1964; Mills, 1969; Niederhoffer, 1967; Rhead, Abrams, Trasman, & Margolies, 1968; Roberts, 1961; Verini & Walker, 1970; Westley, 1956), mentally unfit and cynical (Bain, 1939; Bohardt, 1959; Kates, 1950; Preiss & Ehrlich, 1966; Skolnick, 1966; Westley, 1951; Zion, 1966), corrupt (Smith, 1965; Steffens, 1931; Stern, 1962; Westley, 1951), prejudiced (Banton, 1964; Bayley & Mendelsohn, 1969; Black & Reiss, 1967; Calame, 1970; Ferdinand & Leichterhard, 1970; Henssenstamm, 1971; Kelly & West, 1973; Piliavin, 1973; Preiss & Ehrlich, 1966; Sayre & Kaufman, 1960; Schleifer, Derbyshire, & Martin, 1968; Sikes, 1971; Skolnick, 1966; Wallach, 1970; Westley, 1970), of low intelligence (Bain, 1939; Terman, Otis, Dickson, Hubbard, Norton, Howard, Flanders, & Cunningham, 1917; Thurstone, 1922), less masculine (Terman & Miles, 1936), suicide prone (Niederhoffer, 1967), authoritarian (Carlson, Thayer, & Germann, 1971; Leiren, 1973; Marshall & Mansson, 1966; Matarazzo et al.,

1964; Trojanowicz, 1971; Walther, McCune, & Trojanowicz, 1973), incompetent (Johnson & Gregory, 1971; Rotter & Stein, 1971), motivated to maintain the status quo (Astor, 1971; Bayley & Mendelsohn, 1969; Dodd, 1967; McGaghy, 1968; Niederhoffer, 1967; Walther et al., 1973) and prone to hypochondriasis, compulsive ritual, and the unwarranted abuse of power (Niederhoffer, 1967).

In contrast to the above findings, there are also many positive evaluations of police personality using both psychometric (Blum, 1964; Fenster & Locke, 1973a; 1973b; 1973c; Gottesman, 1969; Guller, 1972; Hogan, 1970; Matarazzo et al., 1964; Mills, 1969; Smith, Locke, & Walker, 1967; 1968; Smith, Locke, & Fenster, 1970; Walther, 1969) and clinical (Lefkowitz, 1971; 1975; Symonds, 1970) procedures.

While much writing about police is speculative and unfounded and while faulty research designs account for much of the confusion (for detailed discussion of this point; see Fenster, Wiedemann, & Locke, 1977), it is most important to distinguish between the *applicants* for criminal justice positions and those who are finally accepted. While there is evidence (Berman, 1971) that maladjusted and otherwise unsuitable candidates often apply for positions in the criminal justice field, very strict procedures for screening police applications exist in almost all major cities. For example, in New York City fewer than 15 percent of those applying for positions as police officers have been accepted (Ellbert, McNamara, & Hanson, 1961; Murphy, 1965; Niederhoffer, 1967); figures are even lower in other jurisdictions (Bohardt, 1959; Matarazzo et al., 1964; Reiser, 1972; Wilson, 1968).

When direct comparisons were made between large groups of police and nonpolice citizens, after methodologic errors had been eliminated police on the whole scored lower on neuroticism, higher in intelligence and (for males) so-called masculinity, and lower in dogmatism. In addition, *college-educated* police were highest in achievement, dominance, and intraception and lowest in nurturance. Noncollege police were distinctive mainly in terms of strong heterosexuality (Fenster et al., 1977). Lefkowitz (1975) had earlier hypothesized that differences between police and nonpolice occur in type of motivation and type of personality rather in degree of psychopathology. Walther (1964) found that policemen valued *standards of authority* (rather than the person who is the authority) and were competitive, assertive, conservative, and oriented toward outdoor and mechanical activities. While there can be no doubt that the criminal justice system in America leaves much to be desired, it is important to distinguish police officers from the system of which they are part. The distinguished psychoanalyst Karl Menninger (1968) writes,

> I have no charges to make against the police as individuals. They do their jobs as they learn them. They are not themselves criminal any more (or any less) than the rest of us. I consider them just as good as I am and I know many of them to be truly superior individuals. What I would point out is that they are trying to do an impossibly

difficult job. They are caught in an obsolete, ineffective, crime-breeding rather than crime-preventing system, which we have inherited. My charges are against the system not the people in it. The system is ours as much as theirs.*

Consulting psychologists must continue to have good reality testing. They must not automatically see police as unjust and oppressive, as minority members often do because police are not visible in the ghetto (Dog, 1968). Even if one concedes that aggression may be an innate drive (Storr, 1968), one must be careful not to project surplus aggression onto police because of their aggressive symbols of gun, nightstick, and uniforms. Negative attitudes toward authorities are learned early in life and are often displaced onto the police. If these authority conflicts are not resolved in consulting psychologists, they are likely to bring negative biases or ''negative counter-transferences'' to the job. These faulty transference attitudes on the part of our citizenry are substantial roadblocks to easing police−community tensions, a problem for which no short-term solutions appear in sight (Wilson, 1968).

Selection and Placement of Police Officers

''Selection'' refers to a decision as to whether or not to hire a police officer; ''placement'' refers to the kind of training or job that an individual police officer will be given (Anastasi, 1968). Consulting psychologists are more frequently than ever before involved in setting up selection procedures involving psychological tests as well as interviews.

We agree with the Task Force Report (1967) that ''complexity inherent in the policing function dictates that officers possess a high degree of intelligence, education, tact, sound judgment, physical courage, emotional stability, impartiality and honesty.''

It is obvious that criteria for selection of police are not absolute and eternal but are relative and everchanging with cyclic variations in economic, political, and social conditions (McManus, 1970). Cutoff scores on tests will be continually revised based on the job market, the individual police department's particular requirements, and feedback from the selection process itself. Setting selection criteria requires the joint wisdom of senior police administrators and consulting psychologists familiar with police organizations.

Overall screening procedures in large cities typically involve a written Civil Service test, a thorough physical examination, a background investigation, and psychological testing. Psychological tests commonly employed are the Minnesota Multiphasic Personality Inventory (MMPI), Rorschach, Thematic Apperception (TAT), Draw a House-Tree-Person, and group intelligence tests, and a short psychiatric interview procedure is also commonly used, with the aim of screening out candidates who are emotionally too disturbed for policework. More recently there has been movement to combine projective

*From Menninger, K. *The crime of punishment*. New York: Viking Press, 1968.

tests such as the Rorschach with more objective standardized measures such as the MMPI and a clinical interview. No attempt is made to find the "ideal police personality," since a variety of healthy personality types are all suited to police work. For example, contrary to the idea that screening should eliminate overaggressiveness, it is probably more essential to eliminate male inadequate personality types who might require institutional backing in order to express their masculinity. For the public this would mean an irresponsibly aggressive police officer. This is just an example of areas needing intensive research.

There is a lack of consensus on several key issues regarding psychological testing of police officers. There is much dispute as to whether selection criteria should be tailored to individual police departments or whether particular standards should apply to varying communities on a citywide, statewide, or even nationwide basis. Another issue is how comprehensive a testing battery is required, since psychological evaluations can be quite expensive. Another potentially explosive problem is how to recruit and select police officers from minority groups. While questions of value are interwoven with questions of efficiency when these problems are raised, much research is necessary to determine, for example, if culture-free or culture-fair tests that ensure competence while not discriminating against minority group members are possible. Similarly, questions as to the optimal amount of psychological testing or the geographic boundaries within which a set of selection criteria should apply can gain much from good psychological experimentation. This is why we feel that ability at research design is such a valuable skill for the psychologist-consultant to possess.

While work is beginning to be carried out in terms of psychological applications to the selection process, more work needs to be done in terms of placement and vocational guidance. Each individual police officer should be counseled in terms of particular strengths and weaknesses determined from psychological tests and interviews, and assignments to specialized jobs should be based more on the basis of an individual's unique talents and abilities than on secondary considerations such as personal influence.

The consulting psychologist should be aware that there may be unhealthy reasons for candidates wanting to become police officers (Berman, 1971). For example, a student recently told one of the authors, "I want to become a cop so that I can shoot down punks." Becoming a police officer may represent an attempt to sublimate aggression and express it in a socially acceptable manner. However, maladjusted individuals who make this attempt may lack proper judgment and ego controls to contain their aggression and channel it properly. Such maladjusted individuals are then more likely to shoot guilty (or even innocent) people unnecessarily and to use undue force or make unnecessary arrests. Similarly, one must be aware of the possibility that males who feel uncertain about their masculinity might (perhaps unconsciously) feel attracted to the gun, club, and uniform. One must also beware of power-hungry individuals eager to dominate others and gratify their egos at the expense of the citizenry they were hired to help. Also, a conscienceless, psychopathically oriented individual might seek to exploit the system and cause many problems. We feel the above illustrations are exceptions rather than the rule partly because thorough selection procedures are used in most instances.

SETTING UP TRAINING PROGRAMS

Consulting psychologists may teach or design courses for training police recruits in human relations, basic psychological aspects of mental health and emotional illness, sexual deviation, juvenile delinquency, principles of counseling, etc. Psychologists should be very concerned about teaching techniques and how the program is presented. One author participated in a teaching program wherein police recruits were sent to a college for academic courses; surprisingly, there were marked behavioral problems in almost all of the classes. Investigation of the situation revealed that there were many factors leading to the breakdown—and most of these factors were operative before the classes even began. First, the students were given no preparation as to what was going to take place. On the day of the first class the students were told about the program and asked to report to the college. The police students were separated from other college students even though they were taught only traditional academic subjects in this program. Interviews with the students revealed marked resentment and confusion on their part. They felt that the higher echelons of the police department were passing the buck by sending recruits to college, indicating that they thought that administrators were afraid that if police officers were accused of showing poor judgment or improper behavior during race riots or campus upheavals the administrators would be criticized and held responsible. The recruits felt that administrators thought they could "pass the buck" to the college by saying, "We provided them with college courses—so if they behave improperly go blame the college!" Students said that middle management personnel (e.g., the sergeants who sat in class with the men they regularly supervised) were very frightened by these new developments, afraid that younger, more educated men would replace them because they had little education. Consequently, the students reported that their sergeants encouraged them to misbehave, insult the teacher, and generally undermine the program. Students felt that the college administration also helped sabotage the program by segregating police recruits into separate classes apart from the rest of the student body and by providing a young and inexperienced part-time, poorly paid, undertrained, and undereducated group of junior faculty to teach them. Subsequent efforts by both the college and the police department helped remedy these difficulties, and the program eventually became quite successful.

In addition to didactic classes, small-group discussions, confrontation situations, sensitivity training, films, role-playing, and videotape feedback are used. Key emotional issues such as feelings about police officers, policework, and minority groups and ways of dealing with difficult street situations all must be discussed. It is important that courses and training manuals not be too "stuffy" and idealistic. All too often, when newly trained recruits begin work and come in contact with their senior colleagues they are told to forget everything they learned at the academy and begin to learn to relate to the real world. Senior police officers should participate in field work training of recruits very early so that the training experience is made relevant and useful.

During training, recruits will be given training in dealing with crisis situations such as suicides, family situations, or crises involving the mentally ill. Recruits should visit a mental hospital and be taught about referral sources in the community for psychological, legal, economic, and medical aid. Bard (1967, 1969, 1970) made a creative innovation when he trained a special unit of the New York City Police Department to handle family disputes. Reiser (1972) feels that such specialization is useful only in geographic areas with high population density. Other interesting experimental approaches to training have been reported by the Metropolitan Police Department (1971), Glaser (1970), Newman & Steinberg (1970), and Sikes & Cleveland (1969). The brochure entitled Mental Illness and Law Enforcement (Burger, 1970) is an excellent attempt to promote constructive interaction between the police and the mentally ill. In New York City 350 hours of the 910-hour training program are devoted to instruction in interpersonal relations (Wetteroth, 1971).

Recruit training must also alert future police officers to the problems they are likely to encounter on and off the job. Spouses of police officers often experience great difficulty in adapting to the special stresses of police work involving unusual and rotating hours, constant threat of their spouse's exposure to danger and death, and overtime requirements without foreknowledge. Male police officers, like many males in our society but perhaps even more so, may have strong needs to prove their masculinity. The male officer provoked by a male suspect trying to prove his own masculinity should not fall into the trap; rather, he should be able to say, "This is not my problem, it is his problem. I know that I am a man, so I don't have to prove it to him." Needless to say, the police officer should not endure physical attack or abuse, and the attacker should be contained—but with the minimum force necessary.

Basic to our viewpoint of facilitating task-oriented behavior from police officers is the need to have police officers understand that early childhood factors will account for much of the irrationality they will observe. Because of their authority role, they will experience an especially heavy dosage of bizarre reactions—most notably unwarranted anger and fear. Thus brazen lawyers may be unable to utter a word when receiving a ticket, and a person's unjustified anger at a police officer may unconsciously represent the anger toward the parent of childhood who caught the person stealing, soiling, or masturbating. Lawbreakers often unconsciously are looking for punishment and wish to be caught, while some masochistic individuals will provoke police officers with taunts and obscenities into hitting them. Similarly, many accidents are motivated by unconscious masochism. A woman who flirts with a male police officer in order to avoid a ticket may be trying to manipulate him just as she manipulated her father as a little girl. Also, unfortunately, it is probably true that the only thing some lawbreakers can accept is force, since as children their parents beat them to make them obey. Early childhood experiences make many criminals seem incorrigible. Police officers must control their own irrational responses, based on their own childhoods, if they are to be maximally effective (Schlossberg & Freeman, 1974). Related to this are the difficulties police officers sometimes have in admitting to or seeking help for emotional problems. Training programs must legitimize the notion that having emotional and physical problems is part of the human experience and is not a sign of decreased masculinity or human failure. Recruits should be informed of resources within the department and within the community that are available for present or future use.

Police psychologists are also involved in training middle management as well as the top management of the police department. Middle management people (e.g., sergeants and lieutenants) often feel trapped between their desires to impress upper-level management and to retain the affection and trust of subordinates. The good middle manager is problem-oriented without a need to dominate or control others, without feeling threatened by the successes of subordinates, and without feeling involved in a popularity contest.

It is becoming more widely recognized that supervisors consciously or unconsciously perform many counseling functions and hence should be given some training in behavioral signals of emotional upset, making referrals, and helpful counseling techniques.

Reiser (1972) says that supervisors should be made aware of the following warning signs of emotional upset:

(a) Drastic behavior change, withdrawal, emotional outbursts, chronic fatigue and irritability, (b) chronic marriage or family problems, (c) depression—talk of quitting or committing suicide, (d) excessive drinking—alcohol on breath often, (e) sexual problems, (f) excessive altercations, (g) accident prone—physical or traffic accidents, (h) physical complaints—headache, backache, stomach pains and others, (i) feeling picked on or misunderstood, (j) deterioration in work performance, (k) loss of self-confidence or interest in job, (l) frequent short-term absences without justification, (m) inability to get along with partners and others, (n) financial problems and outside complaints in the department.*

Problems of suicide, psychosis, or homicidal inclinations all require immediate referral, as do long-standing problems of a chronic nature. It is best for the referral to be voluntary if the supervisor can successfully deal with the police officer's resistance. The consulting psychologist, or other therapists in the community, should be available for consultation or treatment of police officers and their families.

The importance of directness, honesty, informality, establishing rapport, empathetic listening, and reflection of feeling are important principles of counseling and making referrals. Similarly, criticizing, moralizing, or paternalistic or maternalistic behavior on the part of the therapist are to be avoided. A preliminary study has shown the value of training supervisors in the counseling process (Sokol & Reiser, 1969).

Chiefs of police and other top management persons will find that many problems arise out of their authority roles with little or no personal contribution on their part. Workers will feel ambivalent toward "big daddy," at times showing fierce loyalty and at other times showing intense resentment. This is similar to the "transference" relationships that patients develop to their therapists, which often alternate between positive and negative, and is also related to the ambivalence that followers often feel toward their leaders. These problems can be substantially alleviated by developing an open communication system within the Police Department with as much contact as possible between personnel at the top and those at the bottom of the organizational hierarchy. Top management experiences stress from the competing interests in the police organization as well as from rival outside interests in the community. Since not everyone can be pleased, hard choices must be made. Top management training seminars need to focus on ways of assessing the strength and weakness of their organization, personal goals, and self-evaluation. In general there should be much overlap between what a police organization says it does to the community, what it believes it is doing, and what it actually does (Reiser, 1972).

Community relations. In the last 15 years there has been growing tension between police departments and the communities they serve. Situations have sometimes been so explosive that acts (real or imagined) on the part of individual police officers have been said to have triggered off community-wide conflagrations. Niederhoffer (1967) reported that police actions provoked a series of racial disturbances in Harlem, Newark, Philadelphia, Rochester, and Watts.

Consulting psychologists may be involved in designing surveys to tap

*From Reiser, M. *The police department psychologist.* Springfield, Ill.: Charles C. Thomas, 1972.

community and police sentiment on critical issues, they may help design programs designed to foster good police—community relations, and they may conduct encounter groups and sensitivity training for community relations personnel or administrators. Much research needs to be done in this area. Psychologists will also be called on to train detectives and police officers in various specialties that rely heavily on psychological understanding; e.g., interrogating suspects and questioning witnesses. Examining and evaluating scenes of such crimes as homicides and the meaning of evidence gathered after sex crimes may require psychological input.

Homicides. Consulting psychologists are often asked to help solve bizarre murders where the psychological dynamics are of obvious importance. The task of the consultant is to interpret unconscious motives in such a way that an apparently senseless murder (often involving a sex crime as well) will make sense. This kind of activity requires an understanding of personality dynamics, especially the relationships of sex, aggression, and suicidal and homicidal impulses, the unconscious significance of various weapons, and the role of cultural, educational, socioeconomic, occupational, and situational factors. Thus far systematic good research is lacking in this area, although clinical intuition has at times been remarkable. For example, during the height of the police investigation of the ''Mad Bomber'' case, Brussel (1968) said,*

I went on to explain my reasoning about the[Mad] Bomber's personal habits, his paranoiac avoidance of visible flaws. ''He goes out of his way to seem perfectly proper, a regular man. He may attend church regularly. He wears no ornament, no jewelry, no flashy ties or clothes. He is quiet, polite, methodical, prompt. . . . Education: at least two years of high school. The letters seem to show that. They also suggest that he's foreign-born or living in some community of the foreign born. . . . He is a Slav . . . . One more thing,'' I said with my eyes closed tight, ''when you catch him—and I have no doubt you will—he'll be wearing a double-breasted suit.'' ''Jesus!'' one of the detectives whispered. ''And it will be buttoned,'' I said.

After the ''Mad Bomber,'' George Metesky, was caught and hospitalized, Brussel (1968) wrote,

On one of my visits [to Matteawan State Hospital], I had the Mad Bomber brought to the office I used. He was the picture of health; he was calm, smiling and condescending. He was not wearing hospital garb as most patients did. Not George Metesky. He wore his double-breasted suit, and it was buttoned. In the hospital, he was a model inmate, complied with all orders, went to church regularly. . . .

Crisis intervention and on-the-scene assistance. Consulting psychologists may train police in handling of family disputes, crowd control,

*From Brussel, J.A. *Casebook of a crime psychiatrist.* New York: Dell, 1968.

suicide prevention, and hostage situations or may be themselves called to the scene.

In dealing with crisis situations and in solving dramatic crimes, psychologists can actually witness research efforts come to life and assist in solving crimes. Principles of social psychology can be applied by police to control crowds by means other than brute force, and hostage crisis intervention techniques—which have achieved worldwide acclaim for their effectiveness—have drawn on social psychological research efforts in areas such as food and sleep deprivation, response to boredom, need for affiliation, and role expectations (Fenster et al., 1976; Schlossberg, 1974).

Internal affairs. The department of internal affairs investigates charges of misconduct against police officers. The psychologist is often asked to evaluate the police officer in question in terms of emotional stability, ability to carry a gun, etc.

Vice. Consulting psychologists may be called upon to testify as expert witnesses on pornography. They must be familiar with questions of case law, community standards, redeeming social value, and research on the effects of erotic material on children, adolescents, and adults. While current focus has been on paying less attention to victimless crimes (Smith & Pollack, 1971), psychologists are still called upon to testify on questions of vice and pornography.

RESEARCH ROLES OF CONSULTING PSYCHOLOGISTS

The need for systematic planned research in police work has been recognized for some time (Report on Police, 1931; Reddin, 1966; Report of the National Advisory Commission on Civil Disorders, 1968). The police department as well as much of the criminal justice system maintains a policy of official silence amounting to secrecy against disclosure of information (Fenster et al., 1975; Symonds, 1974; Task Force on Police, 1967). More social research is necessary, since the average patrol officer spends more time dealing with human problems and social service than fighting crime (Singer, 1970). New federal funding has acknowledged the need for more police research (L.E.A.A., 1968). An important function of the consulting police psychologist is to help management determine exactly what the in-house research needs are (Kerlinger, 1967). In designing police research, use must be made of the untapped knowledge of experienced police officers as well as the knowledge and techniques of behavioral scientists (Task Force Report on Police, 1967).

More research is needed on the limits of eyewitness perception and recall; Marshall (1966) refers to this as "make-believe evidence," and Brodsky (1972) says, "To paraphrase Santayana, people believe what they see. The problem is they are better at believing than they are at seeing."

"Police intuition" has been called into question by a study (Verinis & Walker, 1970) that showed that police officers who made fewer criminal interpretations were rated by their superiors as more capable than subjects who made more criminal interpretations. More psychological research is needed in the area of perception and criminal investigation.

The recent emphasis on hypnosis as a tool for police work serves as an example of a technique that has been resurrected and reapplied in a new way. Many problems always accompany these innovations, and it becomes the role of the psychologist to explore them for the police department.

There is some question as to whether part-time or full-time psychological consultants are more effective (Reiser, 1972; Shellow, 1971), and this question is itself susceptible to research investigation. More research needs to be done on the selection of law enforcement personnel. In many jurisdictions physical strength and aggressiveness are still the main standards for the selection of police (Task Force on Police, 1967). Narrol and Levitt (1963) reported in a survey of 55 large cities that all were using some kind of psychological test for screening purposes. Research is needed to deal with the difficulties encountered in arriving at consensual standards to predict police personality (Blum, 1964; Smith, 1971). Gottesman (1969) found that the MMPI is of very limited value in selecting police, and Mills (1968) has written about the special problems presented to the psychological evaluation team by police using the rule-of-thumb guide, "if we *all* like him so well, then he can't be much good as a police officer."

Some encouraging beginning research has been done in training police as counselors (Metropolitan Police Department, St. Louis, Missouri, 1971). Also, various new procedures for training police were innovative and appear useful (Bard 1969; 1970; Barocas, 1971; Danish & Brodsky, 1970; Ferguson, 1970; Mills, 1968; Newman & Steinberg, 1970; Rubin, 1970; Siegel, Federman, & Schultz, 1963; Sikes & Cleveland, 1969; Wetteroth, 1971). Research efforts that are interdisciplinary are most likely to be productive (Brodsky, 1976).

In the past there was little interaction between psychologists and police departments; police tended to view psychologists as unrealistic dreamers, while psychologists would view police as Neanderthals (Schlossberg, 1975). Cities such as Los Angeles and New York have begun to hire psychologists on a full-time basis, and the New York City Police Department has one of the nation's first full-time, full-service psychological units, a model for other units that are being created (Fenster et al., 1976; Reiser, 1972; Schlossberg & Freeman, 1974).

REFERENCES

Anastasi, A. *Psychological testing* (3rd ed.). New York: MacMillan, 1968.

Astor, G. The New York cops. *The New York Post*, June 19, 1971.

Bain, R. The policeman on the beat. *The Scientific Monthly*, 1939, *48*, 452.

Banton, M. *The Policeman in the community*. New York: Basic Books, 1964.

Bard, M. Family intervention police teams as a community mental health resource. *Journal of Criminal Law, Criminology and Police Science*, 1969, *69*, 247–250.

Bard, M. *Training police as specialists in family crisis intervention*. Washington, D.C.: U.S. Government Printing Office, 1970.

Bard, M. & Berkowitz, B. Training police as specialists in family crisis intervention: A community action program. *Community Mental Health Journal*, 1967, *3*, 315–317.

Barocas, H. A. A technique for training police in crisis intervention. *Psychotherapy: Theory, Research and Practice*, 1971, *8*, 342–343.

Bayley, D. H., & Mendelsohn, H. *Minorities and the police: Confrontation in America*. New York: Free Press, 1969.

Berman, A. MMPI characteristics of correction officers. Paper presented at Eastern Psychological Association, New York City, April 16, 1971.

Black, D. J., & Reiss, A. J., Jr. Patterns of behavior in police and citizen transactions. In *Studies of crime and law enforcement in major metropolitan areas* (Vol. 2). Washington, D.C.: U.S. Government Printing Office, 1967.

Blum, R. *Police selection*. Springfield, Ill.: Charles C. Thomas, 1964.

Bohardt, P. H. Tucson uses new police personnel selection methods. *FBI Law Enforcement Bulletin*, 1959, *28*, 8–12.

Brodsky, S. L. Special applications to law enforcement. In S. L. Brodsky (Ed.), *Psychologists in the criminal justice system*. Urbana: University of Illinois Press, 1973.

Brodsky, S. L. Psychology and criminal justice. In P. J. Woods (Ed.), *Career opportunities for psychologists: Expanding and emerging areas*. Washington, D.C.: American Psychological Association, 1976.

Brown, W. P. *A police administration approach to the corruption problem*. New York: State University of New York, 1971 (NTIS No. PB 218 936).

Brussel, J. A. *Casebook of a crime psychiatrist*. New York: Dell, 1968.

Burger, K. (Ed.) *Mental illness and law enforcement*. St. Louis: Washington University Social Science Institute, 1970.

Calame, B. E. Man in the middle. In W. H. Hewitt & C. L. Newman (Eds.), *Police-community relations: An anthology and bibliography*. Mineola, N.Y.: Foundation Press, 1970.

Carlson, H., Thayer, R. E., & Germann, A. C. Social attitudes and personality differences among members of two kinds of police departments (innovative vs. traditional) and students. *Journal of Criminal Law, Criminology, and Police Science*, 1971, *62*, 564–567.

Clark, J. P. Isolation of the police: A comparison of the British and American situations. *Journal of Criminal Law, Criminology, and Police Science*, 1965, *56*, 307–319.

Danish, S. J., & Brodsky, S. L. Training of policemen in emotional control and awareness. *American Psychologist*, 1970, *25*, 368–369.

Dodd, D. J. Police mentality and behavior. *Issues in Criminology*, 1967, *3*, 47–67.

Ellbert, L., McNamara, J., & Hanson, V. *Research on selection and training for police recruits: First annual report*. New York: American Institute for Research, 1961, p. 6.

Fenster, A. New forensic psychology M.A. program begun at John Jay College. *American Psychology–Law Society Newsletter*, 1976, *8*, 13–14.

Fenster, C. A., Faltico, G., Goldstein, J., Kaslow, F., Locke, B., Musikoff, H., Schlossberg, H., & Wolk, R. Careers in forensic psychology. In P. Woods (Ed.), *Career opportunities for psychologists*. Washington, D.C.: American Psychological Association, 1976, pp. 123–151.

Fenster, C. A., Litwack, T. R., & Symonds, M. The making of a forensic psychologist: Needs and goals for doctoral training. *Professional Psychology*, 1975, *10*, 457–467.

Fenster, C. A., Litwack, T. R., & Symonds, M. A model for a doctor of psychology program in forensic psychology: Curriculum and rationale. *Teaching of Psychology*, 1976, *3*, 84–88.

Fenster, C. A., & Locke, B. The "dumb cop": Myth or reality? An examination of police intelligence. *Journal of Personality Assessment*, 1973, *37*, 276–281 (a).

Fenster, C. A., & Locke, B. Neuroticism among policemen: An examination of police personality. *Journal of Applied Psychology*, 1973, *57*, 358–359 (b).

Fenster, C. A., & Locke, B. Patterns of masculinity-femininity among college and non-college oriented police officers. An empirical approach. *Journal of Clinical Psychology*, 1973, *29*, 27–28 (c).

Fenster, C. A., Wiedemann, C. F., & Locke, B. Police personality: Social science folklore and psychological measurement. In B. D. Sales (Ed.), *Psychology in the legal process*. New York: Spectrum Publications, 1977.

Ferdinand, T. N., & Lucherhard, E. G. Inner-city youth, the police, the juvenile court, and justice. *Social Problems*, 1970, *17*, 510–527.

Ferguson, R. F. *Creativity in law enforcement: The Covina field experiment*. San Diego: Institute of Public and Urban Affairs, San Diego State College, 1970.

Gilbert, R. Functions of the consultant. *Teachers College Record*, 1960, *61*, 177–187.

Glaser, D. The sociological approach to crime and correction. *Law and Contemporary Problems*, 1958, *23*, 683–702.

Glaser, E. M. *A program to train police officers to intervene in family disturbances* (Final report for L.E.A.A.). Los Angeles: Human Inter-Action Research Institute, 1970.

Gottesmann, J. *Personality patterns of urban police applicants as measured by the MMPI*. Hoboken: Stevens Institute of Technology, 1969.

Grier, W., & Cobbs, P. M. *Black rage*. New York: Basic Books, 1968.

Guller, I. B. Higher education and policemen: Attitudinal differences between freshmen and senior police college students. *Journal of Criminal Law, Criminology and Police Science*, 1972, *63*, 396–401.

Heussenstamm, F. K. Bumper stickers and the cops. *Trans-Action*, 1971, 32–33.

Hodges, A. How not to be a consultant. *Mental Hygiene*, 1070, *54*, 147–148.

Hogan, R. *A study of police effectiveness*. Washington, D.C.: American Psychological Association, 1970.

Johnson, D., & Gregory, J. R. Police-community relations in the United States: A review of recent literature and projects. *Journal of Criminal Law, Criminology, and Police Science*, 1971, *62*, 94–103.

Kates, S. L. Rorschach responses, strong blank scales and job satisfaction among policemen. *Journal of Applied Psychology*, 1950, *34*, 249–254.

Kelly, R. M., & West, G. The racial transition of a police force: A profile of white and black policemen in Washington, D.C. In J. R. Snibbe & H. M. Snibbe (Eds.), *The urban policeman in transition*. Springfield, Ill.: Charles C. Thomas, 1973.

Kerlinger, F. *Foundations of behavioral research*. New York: Holt, Rinehart & Winston, 1967.

Lefkowitz, J. *Job attitudes of police*. National Institute of Law Enforcement and Criminal Justice, U.S. Department of Justice, 1971.

Lefkowitz, J. Psychological attributes of policemen: A review of research and opinion. *Journal of Social Issues*, 1975, *31*, 3–26.

L.E.A.A. *A united strategy for crime control*. Department of Justice, 1968.

Leiren, B. D. Validating the selection of deputy marshals. In J. R. Snibbe & H. M. Snibbe (Eds.), *The urban policeman in transition*. Springfield, Ill.: Charles C. Thomas, 1973.

Levinson, H. *Executive stress*. New York: Harper, 1970.

Marshall, J., & Mansson, H. Punitiveness, recall, and the police. *Journal of Research in Crime and Delinquency*, 1966, *3*, 129–139.

Matarazzo, J. D., Allen, B. V., Saslow, G., & Wiens, A. N. Characteristics of successful policemen and firemen applicants. *Journal of Applied Psychology*, 1964, *48*, 123–133.

McGaghy, C. H. Cops talk back. *Urban Affairs Quarterly*, 1968, *4*, 245–256.

McManus, G. P., Griffin, J. I., Wetteroth, W. J., Boland, M., & Hines, P. T. *Police training and performance study*. Washington, D.C.: U.S. Government Printing Office, 1970, PR-70-4, Grant No. 339, pp. 75–80.

Menninger, K. *The crime of punishment*. New York: Viking Press, 1968.

Metropolitan Police Department, St. Louis, Missouri. Team counseling of hard-core delinquents, November, 1971.

Mills, R. B. Innovations in police selection and training. Paper presented at the annual Convention of the American Psychological Association, San Francisco, September, 1968.

Mills, R. B. Use of diagnostic small groups in police recruit selection and training. *Journal of Criminal Law, Criminology, and Police Science*, 1969, *60*, 238–241.

Murphy, J. J. Improving the law enforcement image. *Journal of Criminal Law, Criminology and Police Science*, 1965, *56*, 105–108.

Narrol, H. G., & Levitt, E. E. Forman assessment procedures in police selection. *Psychological Reports*, 1963, *12*, 691–693.

The New York Times, "CORE Assails Hogan on Gilligan Case," September 3, 1964, p. 19.

Newman, L. E., & Steinberg, J. L. Consultation with police on human relations training. *American Journal of Psychiatry*, 1970, *26*, 65–73.

Niederhoffer, A. *Behind the shield*. New York: Doubleday, 1967.

Pilliavin, J. *Police-community alienation: Its structural roots and a proposed remedy.* Andover, Mass.: Warner Modular Publications, 1973.

Preiss, J. J., & Ehrlich, H. J. *An examination of role theory: The case of the state police.* Lincoln: University of Nebraska Press, 1966.

Radano, G. *Walking the beat.* New York: World, 1968.

Rankin, J. H. Psychiatric screening of police recruits. *Public Personnel Review,* 1959, *20,* 191–196.

Rapaport, D. *Diagnostic psychological testing* (Vol. 1). Chicago: Yearbook Publishers, 1949.

Reddin, T. Police weapons for the space age. *Police Chief,* 1966, 10–17.

Reiser, M. A psychologist's view of the badge. *Police Chief,* 1970, 24–26.

Reiser, M. The police psychologist as consultant. *Police,* 1971, *51,* 58–60.

Reiser, M. *The police department psychologist.* Springfield, Ill.: Charles C. Thomas, 1972.

Report of the national advisory commission on civil disorders. New York: Bantam, 1968.

Report on police. National Commission on Law Observance and Enforcement (Wickersham). Washington, D.C.: U.S. Government Printing Office, 1931.

Rhead, C., Abrams, A., Trasman, H., Margolies, P. The psychological assessment of police candidates. *American Journal of Psychiatry,* 1968, *124,* 1575–1580.

Roberts, E. F. Paradoxes in law enforcement. *Journal of Criminal Law, Criminology and Police Science,* 1961, *52,* 224–228.

Roe, A. *Psychology of occupations.* New York: John Wiley & Sons, 1956.

Rotter, J. B., & Stein, D. K. Public attitudes toward the trustworthiness, competence and altruism of twenty selected occupations. *Journal of Applied Social Psychology,* 1971, *1,* 334–343.

Rubin, R. *Stress training: Trainer's guide to police experience series.* New York: Film Modules, 1970.

Runkel, P. *The law unto themselves.* Ann Arbor: Planaria Press, 1971.

Sayre, W. S., & Kaufman, H. *Governing New York City.* New York: Russell Sage Foundation, 1960.

Schleifer, C. B., Derbyshire, R. L., & Martin, J. Clinical change in jail-referred mental patients. *Archives of General Psychiatry,* 1968, *18,* 42–46.

Schlossberg, H. Down at the station house; Police with psychologic training. *Modern Medicine,* 1975, *43,* 84–89.

Schlossberg, H., & Freeman, L. *Psychologist with a gun.* New York: Coward, 1974.

Shellow, R. Active participation in police decision-making. Paper presented at the Annual Convention of the American Psychological Association, Washington, D.C., 1971.

Siegel, A. I., Federman, P. J., & Schultz, D. G. *Professional police—Human relations training.* Springfield, Ill.: Charles C. Thomas, 1963.

Sikes, M. P. Police-community relations laboratory: The Houston model .*Professional Psychology,* 1971, *2,*, 38–45.

Sikes, M. P., & Cleveland, S. E. Human relations training for police and community. *American Psychologist,* 1968, *23,* 766–769.

Singer, H. A. The cop as social scientist. *Police Chief,* 1970, 52–58.

Skolnick, J. H. *Justice without trial: Law enforcement in democratic society*. New York: John Wiley & Sons, 1966.

Smith, A. B., Locke, B., & Fenster, A. Authoritarianism in policemen who are college graduates and non-college police. *Journal of Criminal Law, Criminology and Police Science,* 1970, *61,* 313−315.

Smith, A. B., Locke, B., & Walker, W. F. Authoritarianism in college and non-college oriented police. *Journal of Criminal Law, Criminology and Police Science,* 1967, *58,* 128−132.

Smith, A. B., Locke, B., & Walker, W. F. Authoritarianism in police college students and non-police college students. *Journal of Criminal Law, Criminology and Police Science,* 1968, *59,* 440−445.

Smith, A. B., & Pollack, H. Crimes without victims. *Saturday Review,* December 1971, 27−29.

Smith, D. H. Police officer selection: A critical literature review. Paper presented at the Western Psychological Association Meetings, San Francisco, April 1971.

Smith, R. L. *The tarnished badge*. New York: Thomas Y. Crowell, 1965.

Sokol, R., & Reiser, M. *A primary prevention proposal utilizing early warning training and division mental health consultants*. Los Angeles Police Department, October, 1969.

Steffens, L. *The autobiography of Lincoln Steffens*. New York: Harcourt, Brace, 1931.

Stern, M. What makes a policeman go wrong? *Journal of Criminal Law, Criminology and Police Science,* 1962, *53,* 98−99.

Stoddard, E. R. The informal "code" of police deviancy: A group approach to "blue coat" crime. *Journal of Criminal Law, Criminology and Police Science,* 1968, *59,* 210−213.

Storr, A. *Human aggression*. New York: Atheneum Press, 1968.

Symonds, M. Emotional hazards of police work. *American Journal of Psychoanalysis,* 1970, *81,* 217−221.

Symonds, M. Curriculum design for the Psy.D. program in forensic psychology. Paper presented at the annual convention of the American Psychological Association, New Orleans, September 3, 1974.

Task Force on Police. *President's Commission on Law Enforcement and Administration of Justice*. Washington, D.C.: U.S. Government Printing Office, 1967.

Terman, L. M., & Miles, C. C. *Sex and personality: Studies in masculinity and femininity*. New York: McGraw-Hill, 1936.

Terman, L. M., Otis, A. S., Dickson, V., Hubbard, O. S., Norton, J. K., Howard, L., Flanders, J. K., & Cunningham, C. C. A trial of mental and pedagogical tests in a civil service examination for policemen and firemen. *Journal of Applied Psychology,* 1917, *1,* 17−29.

Thurstone, L. L. The intelligence of policemen. *Journal of Personnel Research,* 1922, *1,* 64−74.

Trojanowicz, R. C. The policeman's occupational personality. *Journal of Criminal Law, Criminology and Police Science,* 1971, *62,* 551−559.

Verini, J. S. and Walker, V. Policemen and the recall of criminal details. *Journal of Social Psychology,* 1970, *81,* 217−221.

Wallach, I. A. *The police function in a Negro community.* (2 vols.). McLean, Va.: Research Analysis Corporation, 1970, (NTIS No. PB 196 763).

Walther, R. *Job analysis and interest measurement.* Princeton, Princeton Educational Testing Service, 1964.

Walther, R. The psychological dimensions of work. Mimeograph, 1969.

Walther, R. H., McCune, S. D., & Trojanowicz, R. C. The contrasting occupational cultures of policemen and social workers. In J. R. Snibbe & H. M. Snibbe (Eds.) *The urban policeman in transition.* Springfield, Ill.: Charles C. Thomas, 1973.

Westley, W. A. The police: A sociological study of law, custom and morality. Unpublished doctoral dissertation. University of Chicago, 1951.

Westley, W. A. Violence and the police. *American Journal of Sociology,* 1953, *59,* 34−41.

Westley, W. A. Secrecy and the police. *Social Forces,* 1956, *34,* 354−357.

Westley, W. A. *Violence and the police: A sociological study of law, custom, and morality.* Cambridge, Mass.: M.I.T. Press, 1970.

Wetteroth, W. J. The psychological training and education of New York City policemen. Paper presented at the Annual Convention of the American Psychological Association, Washington, D.C., 1971.

Whelton, C. Cooling the rage of the cop in the street. *The Village Voice,* June 24, 1971.

Wilson, J. Q. Dilemmas of police administration. *Public Administration Review,* 1968, *28,* 407−417.

Zion, S. The police play a crime numbers game. *The New York Times,* June 12, 1966, Section 4, p. 6.

Florence W. Kaslow

7

The Psychologist as Consultant to the Court

Serving as a consultant to the court and to its various categories of personnel is a relatively new role for the psychologist; it is probably accurate to say this is an emerging, nontraditional arena of psychologist functioning that seems to have begun slowly in the early 1960s. An extensive perusal of the literature* revealed comparatively few references to such activities by psychologists. Among the few available works in this area are those by Brodsky (1973) and Brodsky and Robey (1972). Brodsky's ideas are invariably action oriented, and his summary (1972) can serve well as a starting point for this chapter:

> The emergence of the psychologist as an expert witness was seen as part of a broad developmental process, including the experimental replication of key factors in evidence, and the offering of clinical and research consultation to judges. It may be through these expanded and creative uses of professional qualified personnel that behavioral scientists will be better utilized and drawn into judicial functions. (pp. 100−101)

One other important recent work bears mention at this juncture because it marks the beginning of a descriptive literature on the myriad tasks the psychologist is, can be, and should be performing in relation to the legal system (Fenster, Faltico, Kaslow et al., 1976).

What literature exists on this topic has not been integrated. This chapter

*Some of the literature search was conducted by Marion Shapiro, Psy.D. Appreciation is expressed to her for her contribution to this chapter. Additional data were drawn from the author's correspondence with "experts" known to be involved in such endeavors as well as from her own observations, teaching, and practice experiences.

endeavors to do this and also to fill some of the gaps. Traditionally, forensics has been considered by many to be the bailiwick of psychiatry. Probably 90 percent of the literature is written by forensic psychiatrists; since I contend that many of the tasks can be equally well performed by qualified psychologists and that the rationale for and philosophy of contributions to the court system is similar for both professions, the forensic psychiatry literature will be drawn upon.

There are areas in which the clinical psychologist might have a slight edge—for instance, diagnostic testing for evaluative and predictive purposes. A similar advantage may hold true for the psychologist trained in organization development approaches, who can be hired as a consultant on streamlining court procedure or resolving court management and staff interpersonal problems. In other cases, there is probably parity and interchangeability possible between professionals from both disciplines.

The organizing schema in the first and largest portion of the chapter revolves around viable and appropriate roles currently being performed by psychologists as consultants to courts. The next section deals briefly with suggested education and training to ensure knowledge and competence to deliver these services. Reflections and a glimpse into the future will constitute the concluding portion.

FUNCTIONAL ROLES OF THE PSYCHOLOGIST AS CONSULTANT TO THE JUDICIAL SYSTEM

A consultant's role is *advisory* and *collaborative*; consultants have no line power of administrative authority over those with whom they are requested or assigned to work (Kaslow, 1972). There are two types of consultant—the internal or in-house consultant, whose major work is within the institution or organization and who is paid a salary, and the external consultant, who is hired by a firm or agency for a specific task or program on a fee basis. In this chapter it is the external consultant whose services are being addressed, unless otherwise indicated.

The judicial process is divided into three phases—pretrial, trial, and posttrial (after verdict and sentencing). The services of a forensic psychologist may be tapped at any or all stages of the process.

Expert Witness—Criminal Cases

CRIMINAL RESPONSIBILITY AND INSANITY DEFENSE

Perhaps the best-known role and that eliciting greatest trepidation in the psychologist is that of expert witness. In a landmark case, *Jenkins v. United States*, (U.S. Court of Appeals for the District of Columbia Circuit, No. 16,

306, 1972), the defendant was convicted of such charges as housebreaking, assault with attempt to rape, and assault with a deadly weapon. A defense of insanity was used. Three psychologists who had examined the defendant were called to present testimony on his behalf. All testified, based on personal contact with him (two as psychologists at St. Elizabeth's Hospital in Washington, D.C., where he had been hospitalized), review of his case history, and results of psychological test batteries, that on the date the alleged crimes were committed he was suffering from schizophrenia, and two of them stated that the disease and the crimes were "related."

The judge, at the conclusion of the trial, told the jury to disregard the testimony of the psychologists (Allen, Ferster, & Rubin, 1968, p. 168). An appeal to the court in the form of an amicus curiae brief submitted by the American Psychological Association (307 F2d, 637, 1962), was heard by a panel of judges, which then held that the Trial Court had "committed a reversible error in excluding the psychologists' expert opinions." The effect of this amicus curiae brief and the decision of the panel of judges was that the psychologists' legitimacy as an expert witness concerning the existence and effects of mental disease or defect was established.

The major points in the argument advanced in the American Psychological Association brief were as follows:

1. Psychology is an established science. It is a scholarly discipline dealing with human behavior; it utilizes scientific methods of investigation and inquiry and criteria of objectivity and thoroughness.
2. The practice of psychology is a learned profession. Students are carefully screened for admission to graduate programs; such programs are accredited by the American Psychological Association, high criteria are held for faculty in keeping with intraprofessional academic requirements; certification and licensing procedures are utilized to denote competency.
3. A clinical psychologist is competent to express professional opinions upon the existence or nonexistence of mental disease or defect and upon their causal relationship to overt behavior. Diagnosis, therapy, and research constitute the main functions of clinical psychologists. They are highly skilled in administering and interpreting psychological tests as part of their diagnostic assessments. These data about personality and behavior that they are capable of formulating are what the court is interested in obtaining.
4. Experience is the essential legal ingredient of competence to render an expert opinion. It must be shown that any witness, to qualify as an expert, possesses special experience and knowledge in relation to the subject. The clinical psychologist is "fully qualified by both occupational experience and by systematic training to express a professional expert opinion in a criminal case." (p. 162). An earlier case, *People v. Hawthorne*, (1940, 293 Michigan 15, 29, N.W. 205) was cited in which the Supreme Court

of Michigan rejected the argument that only a doctor of medicine should be permitted to offer expert testimony. The earlier opinion declares,

There is no magic in particular titles and degrees and in our age of intense scientific specialization we might deny ourselves the use of the best knowledge available by a rule that would immutably fix the educational requirements to a particular degree.

Clearly then, in both *People v. Hawthorne* (1940) and *Jenkins v. U.S.* (1962) the competency of the psychologist to deliver an expert opinion in criminal cases about issues concerning criminal responsibility under the Durham rule (a so-called humanitarian insanity test for an insanity defense in existence from 1954 to 1972) was established and substantiated [see Brooks (1974), pp. 176–183, for a full discussion on the Durham rule].

Quickly the American Psychiatric Association submitted its own brief disagreeing totally with the court's ruling that psychologists are competent to serve as expert witnesses. Their argument stressed that one must be medically trained in order to diagnose mental disease and that psychologists are doctors of philosophy, not medicine.

This stance in 1962 corresponded with an earlier resolution passed by American Psychiatric Association and endorsed by the American Medical Association (AMA) and American Psychoanalytic Association (1954) that only medical training adequately prepared one to diagnose and practice psychotherapy and that relegated psychologists (and other professional personnel) to contributory roles supervised by physicians whenever questions of diagnosis and treatment of illness were involved.*

Ultimately, briefs of both professional associations were heard by the United States Court of Appeals, District of Columbia Circuit, with Judge David Bazelon presiding (*Jenkins v. U.S., 307* F2d, 637, 1962). He placed the problems in the context of legal considerations governing the reception of expert testimony, indicating that two elements are required. First, the person drawing the inferences from the facts must be "so distinctively related to some science [or] profession . . . as to be beyond the ken of the average layman, and second, the witness must have such skill, knowledge, or experience in that field or calling as to make it appear that his opinion or inference *will probably aid the trier in his search for truth"* [italics added] (Allen et al., 1968, p. 176).

Alluding to a number of earlier judicial decisions, Judge Bazelon stated

*This attitude still prevails and is currently espoused in such bills as one before the Wisconsin legislature to legitimize only medical psychotherapy. Psychologists have increasingly resorted to state legislatures to have freedom of choice bills introduced in order for their patients to become eligible to receive reimbursement from third-party payers (insurance companies). Heretofore, the American Psychiatric Association and the AMA have been able to limit such reimbursement to patients of M.D.'s only.

that the general rule is that anyone shown to possess special knowlege and skill in treating "human ailments" is qualified to offer expert testimony, providing that their learning and training indicate that they are competent to tender an opinion on the specific question under consideration. Furthermore, Judge Bazelon reiterated an earlier pronouncement that "it is not essential that the witness be a medical practitioner" (32 C.J.S. Evidence, 1942), stating that often the holder of a Ph.D. in clinical psychology has had a good deal of training and experience in diagnosis and treatment of mental disorders; he held that the lack of a medical degree should not cause automatic disqualification. Rather, "the critical factor in . . . admissibility is the actual experience of the witness and the probable probative value of his opinion." Whenever the issue arises, the trial judge should assess the qualifications of the particular challenged expert; the judge alone makes the decision. The judge, after concluding that the testimony is admissible, should instruct the jurors that it is their responsibility to determine how much weight should be assigned to said testimony.

COMPETENCY TO STAND TRIAL

There are a multiplicity of situations in which the court is involved in making a determination of someone's competency. Perhaps the best-known aspect is the question of whether or not a person is competent to stand trial. In accordance with due process, anyone charged with a crime is guaranteed a rapid trial and the right to legal counsel. A defendant must be physically present and "intellectually capable of participating in his defense" (Robey, 1965). The court will often ask a psychiatrist *or* psychologist for an advisory opinion about the defendant's competency. A pretrial evaluation of the accused should include a diagnostic workup, assessment of commitability, assessment of mental status at the time the alleged crime was committed, and competency to now stand trial. Reports to the court and/or interrogations on the witness stand should revolve around these factors.

While making such evaluations, clinicians should bear in mind that one can be mentally ill and still competent to stand trial; these two issues must be dealt with separately. Also, all too often the M'Naughten rule of criminal responsibility, which applies to sanity at the time the alleged crime was committed (not at the time of the trial), is erroneously used in relationship to the issue of competency to stand trial (Brooks, 1974, pp. 135–160). One must bear in mind that the defendant adjudged incompetent to stand trial is likely to be committed to a state mental hospital for an indeterminate period of time and still have the threat of the dreaded trial looming in the future. Time spent in a mental hospital is not deducted from the eventual sentence. All too often, the stay at the hospital drags on longer than the time a maximum sentence would have lasted in a prison. Such factors are deeply resented by the committed patient and are not conducive to receptivity to treatment; "Why get better if prison appears to await?"

When evaluating an accused's competency to stand trial, the psychologist should bear in mind that one is legally competent "if he is able to understand the nature of the charge against him and aid counsel in preparing his defense" (Slovenko, 1973, p. 92). Robey offers an excellent *Checklist for Psychiatrists* (1965, p. 618) listing criteria for competency to stand trial. Perhaps sometimes the therapist's most humane contribution to a competency hearing is "to help protect a defendant's right to a speedy trial by preventing unnecessary hospitalization" (Bendt, Balcanoff, and Tragellis, 1973, pp. 1288–1289). At no time should psychologists usurp the role of the legal professional; the objective is to assist in the understanding of the questions raised and the behavior observed and to recommend possible alternative solutions, treatment plans, and appropriate placements (Sabot, 1971, pp. 326–328).

COMPETENCY TO BE A WITNESS

There are other times when someone's competency must be determined and the court may turn to a mental health professional for an expert opinion. The credibility of witnesses might be challenged (in criminal or civil cases) if they seem to the judge or jury to be suffering from severe mental or emotional disturbances. An expert opinion might then be sought by "the trier[s] of the fact to determine the extent they may rely on the testimony of the particular witness." Generally, the rule is that a person is considered competent to be a witness in the absence of facts which vitiate the presumption" (Asch, 1973, p. 254) and if the person's mental faculties are in tact enough to make possible rational testimony about the matter being considered by the court. Whenever possible, a direct examination of the witness should be conducted; to assess competency just by observation of behavior in the stressful courtroom situation can lead to a less-than-accurate diagnosis.

TESTIFYING AT A RAPE TRIAL

Despite these several pronouncements about the validity of expert testimony from qualified clinical psychologists, the controversy still rages; the usual practice of members of the bar is to automatically turn to psychiatrists in both criminal and civil cases. However, throughout the country, as in the Jenkins case, courageous, competent, contemporary psychologists are venturing into court rooms. Ellison (1975, p. 5) was asked, as a psychologist knowledgeable about rape, to testify in the Joan Little trial. Eager to avoid becoming ensnarled as an expert for defense and in presenting findings contradictory to those of another impressive expert for the prosecution, she opted to make her contribution by educating the defense team, and hopefully the larger court, about the relevance of some of the political issues of racism and sexism involved that were being ignored. She and one of the female defense attorneys then defined her locus of expertise as centering in the area of *control*, which is the salient factor differentiating rape from consensual sex. Because in institutions such as prisons, inmates are usually deprived of control over their decisions, schedules and activities, the control is lodged in the staff. Thus an unequal power arrangement is established. This led to the line of reasoning Ellison offered in her testimony—that ''any sex between staff and inmates in a total institution must be seen as rape. . . . Free, informed consent is impossible. The inmate subjected to sex with a staff member can be expected to display the crisis reactions found in all victims of forcible rape.'' Questioning from the attorney provided Ellison with the opportunity to relate that individuals in crisis—like Joan Little—cannot be expected to act rationally; thus Ms. Little's testimony about her own behavior when sex was demanded was consistent, in the expert's opinion, with the behavior of a rape victim.

Little was acquitted, with Ellison and the defense team succeeding in being heard by the court, spectators, press, and reading public. The larger political issues of control and authority in situations of unequal power were brought into the limelight. Thus a new function of the psychologist as expert witness appeared on the horizon—that of educator in sociopolitical, legal, ethical, and psychological issues.

Expert Witness—Civil Cases

BUSINESS AFFAIRS

In civil cases, a person's capacity to manage business, financial, and property affairs may be questioned. When this happens, an ''incompetency proceeding'' is instituted (Asch, 1973, p. 7). The judge may ask a court psychiatrist or psychologist or an external consultant to examine the person and report back. Legally, capacity is defined as the specific ability an individual needs to have in order to execute certain acts and undertakings and for them to be held as binding. Thus when someone's testamentary capacity is challenged by disappointed heirs who contest a will, a postmortem psychiatric or psychological evaluation may be ordered by the court. For a will to be declared invalid, the testator would have to be adjudged to have been insane (Slovenko, 1973, p. 344).

DOMESTIC RELATIONS

Psychologists may receive unexpected calls from attorneys asking them to appear as witnesses on behalf of their clients. A not infrequent situation is that of a mother embroiled in a custody suit against a child's father. The psychologist who is called has previously seen the couple in marriage counseling and believes that to be a witness at all violates professional adherence to canons of confidentiality and also forces the taking of sides, and thus refuses. Soon after a subpoena is received. At this point failure to testify can and has resulted in imprisonment (in re Lifschutz, 1970). The guiding principle evolving from the ''Lifschutz compromise'' (Supreme Court of California, 1970) is that one need reveal only information pertinent to the case at hand. Also, the client, in permitting the lawyer to contact the psychologist, has in some way released the psychologist from the bonds of confidentiality and has nullified the doctrine of privileged communication.

This is only one route to becoming a star witness in a custody case. Sometimes the court asks a psychologist, previously uninvolved in the case, to examine parents and child and make a recommendation as to what disposition would be in the child's best interests [see Goldstein, Freud, & Solnit, (1974) for a lengthy and controversial discussion of custody]. As child advocacy services staffed by attorneys appear on the scene, as happened in the family court of Philadelphia in 1975, the child advocate lawyers also turn to psychologists to conduct assessments and make recommendations in custody cases. This is so not only when parents are battling each other for custody but also when a Department of Public Welfare is petitioning to remove an allegedly abused, deprived, or neglected child from the home or prevent the child's return to a deleterious situation.

Some human service professionals are loath to accept such assignments, believing that such matters do not belong in court. However, the court is where such decisions are made, with or without our assistance (Benedek & Benedek, 1972, p. 831); perhaps it is thus incumbent upon psychologists to contribute their sensitivity and acumen to the court's wisdom.

Other reasons for hesitancy to become involved are fear of having one's methods and conclusions disputed or, conversely, having one's recommendations accepted in toto and being placed in the position of playing God in relation to others' lives; yet who other than a psychologist, psychiatrist, or marital-family therapist is qualified by virtue of education and experience to assess a child's needs at a particular stage of development and make a well-calculated guess as to which of the adults available is most likely to offer effective parenting and be most able to share the child with fewer disagreements with the noncustodial parent?

Sometimes when an existing custody decision is challenged, a psychologist may be ''invited to assist counsel on appeal, whether this be in support of a good decision or in opposition to a poor one'' (Benedek & Benedek, 1972, p. 833). Furthermore, Benedek and Benedek recommend that the behavioral scientist leap at the opportunity to be involved.

Psychologists called in to assist in custody cases might find a good set of guidelines in Michigan's Child Custody Act of 1970 (Public Act No. 91). It defines the "best interests of the child" as the sum total of ten variables—including mental and physical health and "moral fitness" of the competing parents and the "reasonable preference of the child" (if the court deems the child to be of sufficient age to express preference).

There are several other types of cases that can be classified under the heading of domestic relations. For example, in divorce cases the psychologist might be called upon in states that have not passed no-fault divorce laws when one party uses mental cruelty as the grounds on which the divorce is being sought (Bezeredi, 1973). Other situations include cases involving annulments, guardianship, and mental health of a spouse prior to marriage.

TEST LITIGATION

Paul highlights *The Psychologist's Role in Litigation Concerning Test Discrimination* (1974, pp. 32–36). In recent years individuals and groups have turned to the courts "alleging that particular tests discriminate against certain minority groups, consequently depriving some individuals of their rightful opportunities" (Paul, 1974, p. 32). Paul was asked by an attorney to collaborate in a case before the Massachusetts Commission Against Discrimination. The complaint charged that because the Boston Public Schools employed a nonvalidated entrance test, black and Puerto Rican children were discriminated against and were being denied admission to three public schools. Paul conducted a validity study of the entrance examination. He also analyzed the school's racial composition, utilizing school yearbooks and attendance records, to see what changes had occurred subsequent to the introduction of the entrance tests. When called to testify, he had hard data to present in addressing the central questions of the litigation and in suggesting how the tests could be reconstructed to predict more accurately the needed abilities for mastery in those schools. This was a novel and ingenious aproach to a relatively new psycholegal problem, and psychologists might well be encouraged by Paul's experience to venture into such heretofore unexplored terrain.

INJURY AND LOSS OF EARNING POWER

Psychologists who have done a great deal of vocational counseling and know the labor market scene in depth are uniquely qualified to serve as expert witnesses in personal injury cases.

In cases involving vocational matters such as a loss of earning power in the competitive labor market, primary data are derived from professional assessment of preinjury and postinjury types and levels of employability, job hiring specifications and pay schedules, and the prevailing labor market. Secondary effects of injury are the clinical-vocational or psychological impairment that may limit employability or career advancement possibilities or contribute to work interruptions in finding and holding suitable employment. Any of these reduces future earning power.

According to Leshner (1975, p. 14), assumptions of the validity of medical evaluation are the usual basis for vocational evidence. Nonetheless, a 50 percent physical disability can result in 100 percent unemployability in one's former occupation. This is the case, for example, when a carpenter loses a thumb and he is no longer capable of manipulating tools. If original potential earning power can be "reasonably established on the basis of pre-injury health, intelligence, socio-economic background and family patterns," it is possible to correlate predicted loss of earning power with labor market projections and trends, future salary scales, and, where children are involved, "with lifetime earnings projected on probable educational achievement."

TRAFFIC ACCIDENTS

Psychologists are often employed as consultants to offer clinical appraisals of the mental state of a person before and at the time of a traffic accident, particularly regarding a subject's level of fatigue, temperament, degree of psychopathology, and presence or absence of drugs or alcohol in the system at the time of the accident (Howard, 1971, pp. 4−11).

All of the foregoing have to do with variations on the expert witness role. Its dimensions are numerous; its implications gigantic for in many instances such expert testimony contributes to determinations of critical import in a person's life such as whether he'll be committed to a mental institution or be given a prison sentence—thus losing his liberty—or whether he will remain free.

We now shift attention to non-expert witness functions the psychologist may be asked to assume on behalf of the court.

Psychological Assessment

In many court clinics, psychologists conduct presentence evaluations on the basis of which they can make appropriate recommendations to the court regarding case disposition. The use of psychiatric (and psychological) consultation at the point of sentencing is rare. However, signs of change are on the horizon. The Forensic Clinic at UCLA offers consultation to the court at the sentencing phase, and Suarez (1972) suggests that this program can serve as a model. The clinic's agreement with the court is that the clinic will restrict exploration to issues pertinent to sentencing and disposition. Evaluation concentrates on "what is happening in the individual, how the offense fits in this context, [and] what the individual needs in terms of therapy and rehabilitation [including] specific discussion of these needs and the agencies that might meet them" (Suarez, 1972, p. 296). In shifting the emphasis away from the verdict and toward the disposition, resistance has been encountered from judges and lawyers; therefore the clinic staff embarked on an extensive educational program with courtroom personnel. Suarez considers these collaborative efforts to have been fruitful.

In prisons, psychologists are asked to evaluate inmates being considered for parole, pardon, or commutation. Their reports become part of the data on which the judge's or Pardons Board's decision is based.

Frequently a salient question in commitment hearings and in contemplation of parole or pardons revolves around a person's "dangerousness." Prediction of future dangerousness is at best a very inexact and hazardous task and yet one that psychologists are frequently called upon to render. This is increasingly true today, since a person being or remaining committed in many states must now be both mentally ill and dangerous (*Donaldson v. O'Connor*, U.S. Supreme Court, 1975). Possibly the most definitive handling of this topic is Rappeport's *The Clinical Evaluation of the Dangerousness of the Mentally Ill* (1967).

It goes without saying that the battery of tests selected is determined by the reason for the referral and what type of data is sought. As an extreme example, one would utilize a very different battery for testing to make a determination of commitability or competency to stand trial than one would for deciding what kind of treatment plan should be devised. When no suitable test instrument exists, initiative should be taken to see that one is constructed (Fenster, Litwack, & Symonds, 1976, p. 140).

When the issue of commitment arises, the judge or master wants to know why it is essential to deprive someone of their liberty. One reason is that the subject may be dangerous to self as well as to others. Psychologists are uniquely competent to identify overt indicators of potential suicidal efforts, not only from the verbal expression of the ideation, or from knowing the meaning of such behaviors as suddenly giving away valuable possessions and expressing extreme despair (Kaslow, 1975), but also from the more subtle clues appearing in such tests as Draw a House-Tree-Person, Thematic Apperception, and Rorshach.

Treatment

Many juvenile and family courts now have their own clinics, either in court facilities or as nearby satellite centers, offering individual, family, and group therapy to justice clients. Sometimes becoming involved in therapy is made a condition of probation; sometimes it is used as an alternative to probation or detention. Where no court clinic exists, or where additional services are needed, judges send court-mandated referrals to community mental health centers. Increasingly more courts are establishing their own clinics, since they are then assured more rapid service, easy communication, and no refusal of their referrals.

Justice clients are often hostile, furious, impulse ridden, antisocial, and hard to treat; diagnostically many have character or personality disorders (Reiner & Kaufman, 1959) and require great patience and skill from the therapist. The clinical psychologist cognizant of the special dilemmas and needs of the court-mandated-for-treatment clients can serve as a consultant and staff trainer to clinic staff.

Research and Program Evaluation

Some court mental health clinics have developed services for selected groups of clients such as sex offenders; these programs are intertwined with ongoing research with these clients geared to yielding practical data as well as theoretical suggestions for treating pedophiliacs, exhibitionists, and others. Clinics in Philadelphia, Baltimore, and Toronto are currently offering such specialized services (Brodsky, 1973, p. 98).

McGee and Bennett (cited by Brodsky, 1973, p. 99) have made several worthwhile avant garde proposals on ways psychologists can assist judges in understanding relationships among decisions, processes, and outcomes. They indicate that many judges have voiced interest in learning the outcome of decisions they have rendered. Psychologists could thus use their research skills to investigate such matters as length of sentence as a deterrent, subsequent adjustment (in relation to type of sentence meted out), and the nature and impact of complex psychological factors in the courtroom. Although not all judges are ready to become involved in such studies, many are, and the timing seems right for such studies to be undertaken. "Study of the judicial process might include the evaluation of the probability of witnesses' perceptual errors, assessment of the veracity of those testifying, and inquiry into the psychological functioning of juries" (McGee and Bennett, cited by Brodsky, 1973, p. 99). In using social and behavioral science knowledge and methodology to study law and the judiciary, one might well produce material that would be useful in the continuing education of judges.

Case Consultation: An Anecdote

In 1975 it was my good fortune to be invited to serve as a consultant to the Family Court in Tokyo, Japan. The consultee group was composed of marriage counselors on the court's staff and judges, all male. Only one, Mr. S., who had taken some training at the Marriage Council of Philadelphia, spoke any English. Since I speak no Japanese, he served as interpreter. In

Japan, couples experiencing marital discord seek help from the court's counselor-conciliators; if the problems cannot be resolved, they are referred by the counselor to a judge.

Mr. S. had written up on large newprint sheets excerpts from the cases the counselors wished to discuss with me. The four cases presented had a common theme—the wife's inability to be subservient to the husband's parents, with whom they invariably were living. All of the women were products of modern Japan and had worked prior to marriage and achieved a reasonable degree of independence. However, upon marrying, each was expected to conform to the traditions of an earlier period and move in with the husband's parents and cater to their wishes. Refusal to do so was not tolerated; thus a seemingly schizophrenic withdrawal occurred, at which point husband and parents became disenchanted with the quiet, depressed wife and sought counseling. Frequently in such cases a diagnosis of schizophrenia or depression is made and the wife is hospitalized.

In doing consultation for people of another culture, it is of course essential to be mindful of their heritage, traditions, and values. Being careful to preface my case analysis with remarks such as, ''I realize that in Japan this handling is in accord with your family system,'' and attempting to exercise the utmost of tact throughout, it was then possible to introduce another perspective for understanding and treating such cases, one that might be used by marital therapists in the United States.

I raised questions about whether the son might be helped to be more assertive on behalf of the needs and rights of his wife; whether it is still so essential to live with parents and, if not, what differences might be expected in the marital interaction were the couple to live alone; whether the parents' demands or expectations were even dealt with in therapy with an attempt to lessen the authoritarian and total nature of them.

Despite the language barrier, a lively dialogue took place, and there was a real sharing of philosophies about family systems, dynamics, and marital counseling approaches. Cannot similar case consultations be held on difficult cases with court staffs in our own country?

EDUCATION AND TRAINING OF THE PSYCHOLOGIST FOR THESE FORENSIC ROLES

Ideally, doctoral students interested in forensic psychology should be able to specialize in this area. One plan currently under consideration at John Jay College (New York) is a Psy.D. in forensics—a total concentration in both course work and internships (see Fenster, Litwack, & Symonds, 1976, pp. 84-87 for a description of the program). A recent development is the combined Ph.D.–J.D. program. Pioneered at the University of Nebraska Psychology Department and Law School in Lincoln, Nebraska, and under the able direction of Bruce Dennis Sales, Ph.D.–J.D., this program has been underway for several years but has yet to graduate its first students. It is a five year program, admitting five students per year. In the fall of 1979 two more Ph.D.–J.D. programs are scheduled to start. One is between the University of Maryland Law School and John Hopkins University Department of Psychology. The other is a joint program in Pennsylvania between the Department of Psychology Education at Hahnemann Medical College and the Law School at Villanova University. Instrumental in bringing this latter program to fruition, I am convinced that concurrent education in both disciplines is a better model for an integrated understanding of both fields than the sequential model of acquiring one degree and then becoming immersed in the second field of study. Also at Hahnemann, all Psy.D. candidates have, for the past five years, taken courses in treatment in correctional settings and forensic psychology. Field trips during these two courses have included visits to prisons, detention centers, and court hearings to maximize exposure to where and how the events really take place. It is possible for students to select an internship in a criminal justice agency.

Some of the content areas requiring coverage in a forensic education or training curriculum follow.

Confidentiality, Limits to Conifidentiality, and Informed Consent

It is urgent that psychologists know just how far they can guarantee confidentiality and be able to explain to their own patients, as well as to anyone they are examining on behalf of the court, what the limits to confidentiality are. Ideally, this should be done in the first session. The doctrine of informed consent rests on the patient or person being evaluated being in a rational state of mind with sufficient latitude of choice to agree or disagree to a procedure or use of information (Sadoff & Kaslow, 1974).

Familiarity with key legal decisions affecting mental health practice and forensic psychology concerns should be fostered; for instance, students should be familiarized with the Tarasoff case, in which the California Supreme Court (1974) held that "private privilege ends where public peril begins;" that is, a therapist must report to the appropriate authorities or warn the potential victim when a patient is threatening violence and the therapist believes that the contemplated aggressive behavior is likely to erupt. This decision (see A. P. A. Monitor, March 1975) heralds a landmark ruling that may well influence the handling of confidentiality by therapists in many states. It has been dubbed the "duty to warn" law.

Students should be encouraged to think through the ethical and therapeutic implications inherent in confidentiality and dangerousness concerns as well as the multifaceted responsibilities to patient, agency or institution, society, and their own profession.

The Role of the Expert Witness

If the premise advanced earlier—that the well-trained doctoral-level psychologist can and should serve as an expert witness when invited to do so—is accepted, then careful preparations for the complexities of this role should be given.

The psychologist who as a therapist has been seeing the person involved in the trial or hearing should try to anticipate probable questions, come in well prepared and try to adhere to the canon of confidentiality as much as possible, and as discussed earlier, disclose only that information pertinent to the substance of the trial. The psychologist requested by counsel to conduct a diagnostic evaluation must prepare an appropriate report of findings and be able to interpret this clearly in a vocabulary that non-mental health personnel can understand.

Visits to the court to become familiar with the procedure are in order, as are briefing sessions with the attorney. Brodsky and Robey (1972) offer an excellent discussion on how to become a good expert witness and delineate the three phases of a continuum of forensic involvement as (1) pretrial, (2) actual activities on the witness stand, and (3) posttrial. Their main point, that the courtroom-oriented witness is much more effective (and less anxiety ridden), is the reason for including this topic in a forensic course.

Frequently, when expert testimony is solicited from mental health professionals, contradictory expert witnesses will be presented by the opposing sides. Since the legal process in the United States is predicated on an adversary relationship, attorneys perceive themselves as advocates for something or adversaries against it and tend to cast expert witnesses into similar stances. There is continuing debate as to whether expert witnesses can ever truly be idealized, detached, completely neutral persons objectively presenting facts as they see them, which is how most psychologists imagine themselves in such circumstances (Brodsky & Robey, 1972, p. 173). To be such a neutral expert, however, one would have to be functioning outside of the court's traditional adversary system and be neither in the employment of the defense nor of the prosecution. Most expert witnesses are hired and compensated for their services by either defense or prosecution; the truly neutral expert would have to be employed by and to act on behalf of the court, thereby reducing disagreement between expert witnesses for each side and assisting the court in arriving at more fair, impartial decisions. Diamond (1968, p. 145) describes prevailing practice as ''the fallacy of the impartial expert.'' He cites the customary manner of labeling witness as *for* the defense or *for* the prosecution to document the inherently adversary expectation.

Graduate students should be schooled in the psycholegal subtleties involved in the expert witness role and the issue of who one is representing. Queries regarding the psychologist's responsibility to the person paying the fee, to the defendent whose life or liberty may be at stake, to the court, and to the society that mandates its criminal justice system to protect it from the dangerous, and dictates of the psychologist's professional ethics should abound in classroom discussions.

Psychologists must learn how to defend their status as experts and how to handle cross and redirect examinations, since they will have to submit to this and substantiate their own statements whether they appear as impartial, independent, court-appointed witnesses or as adversary witnesses (Diamond, 1968, p. 146). Some authors, such as Kubie (1973), urge that the psychiatrist should not be a witness for either side but rather should be hired either by both sides or by the court. He cites the Ruby case to demonstrate how the adversary system can destroy the validity of a psychiatrist's testimony.

There are no simple, definitive answers about confidentiality, limits to confidentiality, the parameters in which the expert witness operates, or any other aspect of forensics practice. Therein lie the excitement, the professional challenge, and the risks.

REFLECTIONS AND SUGGESTIONS: THE FUTURE IS NOW

In all of the foregoing, an action orientation has abounded; suggestions have been made as to forensic areas in which some adventuresome psychologists are already functioning and which are fertile fields for expanded and more numerous efforts. The following is a nonexhaustive attempt to stimulate movement into new channels where need is great.

Legislators

The law under which the courts operate is derived from two sources, legislative enactments and the body of judicial precedents. Psychologists have played a relatively insignificant part in influencing kinds and content of mental health legislation being introduced and considered and would do well to serve as consultants to state and Federal legislative committees drafting bills on delinquency, substance abuse, abortion, gun control, and sex education as well as on the periodic revisions of mental health and mental retardation acts. Self-interest is not a valid basis for such involvement; concern for the mental health and well-being of the public must be the motivating factor conveyed to legislators.

Probation and Parole Officers

The day-by-day overseeing of the lives of many justice system clients not living in institutions is the jurisdiction of court-related probation and parole staff. They check to see that the conditions of probation are being met, assist the clients in improving their capabilities and the quality of their lives, and aid the client in efforts to "go straight." Many of these staff members have bachelor degrees; increasingly more departments are hiring those with M.S.W.'s and M.A.'s. In some cities, such as Philadelphia, probation departments maintain special service units with staff serving as therapists, yet many social workers and psychologists face a dilemma in that they "feel that case work [and psychotherapy*] cannot be effectively offered in an authoritative agency;" they have been indoctrinated with a belief that authority interferes with treatment, since the latter can occur only "in an aura of permissiveness, acceptance, support and self-determination" (Main, 1972, p. 190). Some workers are capable of rehabilitation counseling and therefore resent being pushed to make referrals to mental health agencies, yet they question the efficacy of treatment when it is mandatory. The psychologist-consultant can make a tremendous contribution in areas such as helping parole and probation staff with their identity problems and expanding their dynamic understanding of the client population and case management.

Selection of Jurors

Surprisingly, little literature is to be found about this topic. Assuming that jurors are supposed to be capable of making rational decisions based on the ability to comprehend the evidence being presented and witness credibility, it is my belief that they should possess some minimal level of intelligence, be unbiased and invulnerable to pressure, and be in reasonably sound mental health. Psychologists could devise a more standardized screening procedure and participate in implementing the process, particularly if a jury is being selected for a well-publicized or potentially controversial and explosive trial such as that of the "Chicago Eight."

In late 1976 I was asked to serve in a consultant capacity to a defense attorney in jury selection for a case being tried in a Federal district court. Because of the subtlety and complexity of the issues involved and the potentially long sentence that might be meted out to his client, the attorney knew

*Words added.

that the role of the jury would be a crucial one and was seeking an intelligent and sensitive jury. Together we drew up a preferred profile of the "ideal juror" and worked out a formula for selecting such given the demographic data appearing on the list of potential jurors.

Research and Evaluation

Possibly because of meager budgets and the lack of program evaluators on staff, most criminal justice programs are not subject to rigorous evaluation. Programs are often instituted and perpetuated because someone believes they will help; then vested interests evolve. Consultant psychologists can help develop appropriate study designs, supervise the evaluation process and the analysis and interpretation of data, and relay this to court administrators, who can then better assess program and system effectiveness.

Two particular areas in which a great deal of systematic research is needed are ways of preventing recidivism and accurate assessment tools for predicting dangerousness. Psychologists who could spearhead such research and develop viable techniques would indeed be making a major contribution to society and its well-being.

Institutes for Judges and Attorneys; Courses in Law Schools

Today, with the expanding number of areas in which law and mental health interface, many psychologists have a desire to know more about the laws that govern their practices and the lives of their patients and about the judicial system. Conversely, law students, attorneys, and judges often want to know more about human behavior, motivation, psychodynamics, psychological terminology, understanding psychological test reports, and why and how so much data can be derived from projective tests. Some are amenable to having courses or institutes led by psychologists; this certainly appears to be a valid and attractive field to pioneer. A continuing education course in forensic psychology and psychiatry was offered at Hahnemann Medical College in 1977 to meet such an expressed need.

Special Consultative Services to Judges

Occasionally a judge is confronted by a case that is particularly perplexing and baffling. Some judges find it helpful to talk informally to a sensitive clinician, who can be a sounding board and a generator of additional ideas.

Other judges want help in identifying appropriate community resources. Some want guidance on what gaps exist in the service network, some seek ideas on how to see that needed new programs and facilities are begun.

Psychology and law today interface on many new waves of an uncharted and choppy sea. Little has been said about the myriad problems members of the two disciplines have when they initially encounter each other professionally—problems of vastly different vocabularies and orientations. However, increasingly we need to work collaboratively as the body of mental health law expands and as more of the areas of psychological practice are regulated by law. Since fear of the unknown breeds anxiety and conflict, it is to be assumed that as we become more familiar with the judicial system (and vice versa) we will be more capable of working in tandem when necessary while still maintaining our distinctiveness and our separate functions and values in relation to clients of the justice and mental health systems.

THE AMERICAN BOARD OF FORENSIC PSYCHOLOGY

In 1978 the American Board of Forensic Psychology was founded and incorporated to define the functions of the forensic psychologist, to promulgate standards for this specialization, and to make those in the justice system aware of the numerous psychologists who are competent as forensic specialists. As of January 1979, the board began certifying such experts at the diplomate level.

REFERENCES

Allen, R.G., Ferster, E.Z., & Rubin, J.G. *Readings in law and psychiatry*. Baltimore: Johns Hopkins Press, 1968.

Asch, S.H. *Mental disability in civil practice*. Rochester: Lawyers Cooperative Publishing, 1973, chaps. 1 and 11.

Bendt, R., Balcanoff, E., & Tragellis, G. Incompetency to stand trial: Is psychiatry necessary? *American Journal of Psychiatry*, 1973, *130*, 1288–1289.

Benedek, E.P., & Benedek R.S. New child custody laws: Making them do what they say. *American Journal of Orthopsychiatry*, 1972, *42*, 825–834.

Bezeredi, T. Psychiatric assessment of mental cruelty. *Canadian Psychiatric Association Journal*, 1973, *18*, 273–277.

Brodsky, S. *Psychologists in the criminal justice system*. Urbana: University of Illinois Press, 1973, chap. 9.

Brodsky, S. Consultation to criminal justice agencies: The ambivalent consultee. In S. Plog & P. Ahmed (Eds.), *The art of mental health consultation*. New York: Academic Press, 1976.

Brodsky, S., & Robey, A. On becoming an expert witness: Issues of orientation and effectiveness. *Professional Psychology*, Spring 1972, 172–176.

Brooks, A. *Law, psychiatry and the mental health system*. Boston: Little, Brown, 1974.

Child Custody Act of 1970, Public Act No. 91. *Michigan compiled laws annotated*. St. Paul: West Publishing, sections 722.21–722.29.

Diamond, B. The fallacy of the impartial expert. In R. Allen, E. Ferster, & J. Rubin (Eds.), *Readings in law and psychiatry*. Baltimore: Johns Hopkins Press, 1968.

Ellison, K. Psychologist in court: Testimony on rape in the Joan Little trial. *Social Action and the Law*, 1975, *2* (6), 5.

Fenster, A., Faltico, G., Goldstein, J., Kaslow, F., et al. Careers in forensic psychology. In P. Woods (Ed.), *Career opportunities for psychologists*. Washington, D.C.: American Psychological Association, 1976.

Fenster, A., Litwack, T., & Symonds, M. A model for a doctor of psychology program in forensic psychology: Curriculum and rationale. *Teaching of Psychology*, 1976, *3*, 84−87.

Goldstein, J., Freud, A. & Solnit, A. *Beyond the best interests of the child*. New York: Behavioral Science Book Service, 1974.

Howard, L.R. Forensic psychology and road traffic accidents. *Journal of Forensic Psychology*, 1971, *3*, 4−11.

Jenkins v. United States, Brief for American Psychological Association, amicus curiae U.S. Court of Appeals for the District of Columbia Circuit, No. 16, 306, 1962, and 307 F2d, 637, 1962.

Kaslow, F. *Issues in human services: A sourcebook in supervision and staff development*. San Francisco: Jossey Bass, 1972.

Kaslow, F. Suicide: Causation, indicators and interventions. *Journal of Sociology and Social Welfare*, 1975, *999*, 60−80.

Kubie, L.S. The Ruby case: Who or what was on trial. *Journal of Psychiatry and Law*, 1973, *1*, 475−491.

Leshner, S. Vocational evidence. *Pennsylvania Psychological Bulletin*, April 1975, 14.

in re Lifschutz, 85 Cal. Reporter, 829, 476 P 2d 557 (California Supreme Court, April 15, 1970).

Main, J. Supervision of juvenile court probation officers. In F. Kaslow (Ed.), *Issues in human service*. San Francisco: Jossey Bass, 1972.

Paul, L. The psychologist's role in litigation concerning test discrimination. *Professional Psychology*, February 1974, 32−36.

Rappeport, J. (Ed.). *The clinical evaluation of the dangerousness of the mentally ill*. Springfield, Ill.: Charles C. Thomas, 1967.

Reiner, B., & Kaufman, I. *Character disorders in parents of delinquents*. New York: Family Service Association of America, 1959.

Robey, A. Criteria for competency to stand trial: A checklist for psychiatrists. *American Journal of Psychiatry*, 1965, *122*, 616−623.

Sabot, T. Mental health consultation concerning the competency of the criminal defendant. *Community Mental Health Journal*, 1971, *7*, 323−330.

Sadoff, R., & Kaslow, F. *Confidentiality for psychotherapists working within the criminal justice system* (Position paper promulgated by Pennsylvania Bureau of Correction, 1974; available from author).

Slovenko, R. *Psychiatry and law*. Boston: Little, Brown, 1973.

Suarez, J. Psychiatry and the criminal law system. *American Journal of Psychiatry*, 1972, *129*, 293−297.

Paul Gendreau,
D. A. Andrews

8

Psychological Consultation in Correctional Agencies: Case Studies and General Issues

The rapid growth of psychological services in corrections (Gendreau, 1979; Gormally & Brodsky, 1973) has been paralleled by the development of university-based training programs in correctional work (Andrews & Gendreau, 1976; Fenster, Litwack, & Symonds, 1975; Speilberger, Megargee, & Ingram, 1972). While the degree and range of psychologists' activities has advanced (Brodsky, 1972; Wicks, 1974), much of psychological programming in corrections is still in its infancy. One such example is that of consultation.

Consultation has achieved considerable popularity in mental health and education settings, as indicated by the many descriptions of consultant activity that have appeared in the literature. Proponents of consultation argue that the consultant has the potential to create a greater and more diverse impact on the agency and its clients relative to the model of direct service that psychologists have traditionally adhered to (see Mannino & Shore, 1975). Thus it would

The views expressed in this paper do not represent Ontario Ministry of Correctional Services Policy.

The following individuals have all played important roles in the consultation activities described in this paper: Ernest Bond, Jim Bonta, Andy Birkenmayer, Gerry Brown, Doretta Burke, Robert Cormier, Wendy Daigle-Zinn, Carl DeGrandis, Mac Doraty, Roger Dupuis, John Ecclestone, Colin Farmer, Lorna Gendreau, Brian Grant, Linda Hearst, Flo Hughes, Judith Hughes, Michael Irvine, William Jackson, Frank Kaar, Christine Kennedy, Donald Kennedy, Jerry Kiessling, Roger Kimmerley, Marina Kouri, Leah Lambert, Eino Loukko, Hugh Marquis, Earl Martin, Ray Dev. Peters, Roberta Russell, Wally Schneider, Ash Sial, Syd Shoom, Mort Smyth, Tom Surridge, Stephen Wormith, and Gordon Young.

appear that consultation might be a similarly effective means of initiating the process of change in corrections. Indeed, some have argued (Twain, McGee, & Bennett, 1972) that consultation may be the most useful method of service delivery available to correctional psychologists.

To date, there have been relatively few descriptions of consultation in correctional settings. In contrast to the mental health and education literature, the reported outcomes on correctional consultation are at best mixed, with as many failures being reported in setting up viable services in correctional institutions (Katkin, 1972; Katkin & Sibley, 1973; Repucci, Sarata, Saunders, McArthur, & Michlin, 1973; Sebring & Duffee, 1977) as successes (Bayer & Brodsky, 1972; Gluckstern & Packard, 1977; McDonough & Anderson, 1969; Repucci, Dean, & Saunders, 1975; Repucci & Saunders, 1974). However, general statements of this sort might be premature given that these efforts have taken place in different settings—Attica to small jails—and have involved diverse objectives. In addition, comparative data on consultation efforts in corrections have been nonexistent. A good deal more evidence needs to be collected where factors of general interest in consultation are examined in relation to impact across a range of settings and consultation activities.

We document 19 consultation efforts that took place in 12 correctional agencies ranging from maximum security institutions to small local jails as well as community agencies. Since one or both of the authors were involved in each consultation effort as either consultant or contractor of consultant services, the efforts may be compared in terms of the nature of the setting, the nature of the consultant's activities, and the ultimate impact of those activities.

The majority of the consultation activities described include a formal assessment of the effects of the consultant programs upon the agencies' clients. Also, the impact of consultation on the social and organizational structure of the agencies themselves is examined. In this regard, one of the indices of impact chosen was the survival, maintenance, or continuing development of programs once the consultant exited.

In describing each setting where consultation efforts occurred we chose *not* to organize our description on the basis of consultation models. In our view many of the consultation models (e.g., Caplan, 1970; Schein, 1969) are typologies, and we question how useful a label or typology is in regard to developing actual services. Second, it is difficult to maintain distinctions such as client-centered, consultee-centered, and case-versus-administrative consultation (Korchin, 1976); rather, it has been our experience that the emphasis should be on phases of consultation and that there is no necessary relationship between type of consultation and phase. Moreover, consultants can incorporate three basic elements of applied science that coincide with their activities in each phase—an exploration of the problem and assessment of the controlling variables, the design and implementation of an intervention plan on the basis of the definition of the problem, and an evaluation of the applied value of the program. In effect, the consultant operates as a ''scientist-consultant.''

In our case study descriptions we focus on three common-sense phases in the consultation process—entry, participation, and exit.

Entry. While the entry aspect has been neglected in the consultancy literature (Cherniss, 1976), just how entry is achieved can directly influence the quality of participation. Relevant entry variables are the initiator of the contact, the consultant's preknowledge of the setting, the stability of the inmate and management environment, how the consultant is paid, and the congruence in values, i.e., the functions of correctional settings, treatment versus punishment, etc. between the consultant and the agency administration.

Participation. The important variables at entry also influence problem definitions, the courses of action taken by the consultant, and the indices by which goal attainment are gauged. Furthermore, the degree and range of the consultant's activity are crucial to the participation phase. A standard definition is that the consultant's activity ''enables others to do'' (Caplan, 1970), which in our view is far too limiting (if not unrealistic) as to how the consultant's role may shift dramatically during the participation phase of consultation.

Exit. The entry and participation phases result in at least an informal contract and hence a definition of when consultation comes to an end or when a new contract should be formed. We see three distinct issues in the exit phase—the documentation of programs by formal research reports, program maintenance, and evidence of influences on agencies beyond the host agency.

Finally, we consider crucial the relationships observed across various settings between consultation process variables and the program maintenance factor because the most important result the consultant can hope to achieve is a change in the social and organizational role of the agency so that it better meets the needs of its clients.

CONSULTATION SERVICES

Consultant activities were initiated in 1969 in minimum and medium security institutions, subsequently in jails and regional detention centers, and finally in community-based agencies.

Minimum Security

We have had experience in developing consulting services in a minimum security setting with one institution, Rideau Correctional Centre of the Ontario Ministry of Correctional Services. The institution was generally regarded as a pastoral backwater, with its prime programming feature being a large, mixed farming operation. It had the oldest staff of all Ministry correctional centers; for some it provided part-time jobs. In the late 1960s the institution underwent considerable upheaval with the appointment of professional personnel as well as a superintendent who entered the correctional system from an industrial background. Throughout this period of administrative changes there was little unrest among the residents; in this sense the institution remained stable, as it always had been. Structurally there was also little change. Residents were housed in dormitories and by correctional standards there was virtually no security, i.e., no walls or fences. The population varied from 160 to 220. Most of the residents came from the eastern region of the province, about 40 percent from smaller towns and rural areas. Sentences ranged from one month to two years.

The first set of consultant services operated under a general mandate, i.e., establishment of psychological programs. In contrast, the second consultation program was established in response to a specific management request. The third consultant enterprise grew out of the previous two. The initiation for the first consultant intervention came from the head office and the consultant. The other two consultant programs were initiated locally.

COUNSELING SERVICES

Initially, with the impetus from the new management, it was important to establish a program that would reach a substantial percentage of the residents. In doing so the consultant worked through two distinct planning stages.

The first step was to examine population characteristics and institutional resources (Andrews, Note 1). In 1969, the site was divided into two institutions that shared administrative and professional services. The Training Centre received young (16−21 years old) male first incarcerates and very young (16−18 years old) male recidivists, whereas the Industrial Farm received older male recidivists (19+ years old). The institutions were characterized by very high admission rates (over 800 men per year), a wide resident age range, and a marked variety in current offences and in presenting problems. Inmates at the Industrial Farm also had very short sentences: 83 percent were admitted with a sentence of three months or less and 57 percent were serving sentences of less than 40 days. Even within the Training Centre the actual number of formal training days that residents were available was very low; less than 30 percent of the admissions were present for more than 70 days on which academic, vocational, and counseling programs could be fully scheduled.

At the time that the review of population characteristics was completed, the on-site professional staff included one full-time male nurse, two academic teachers, three shop instructors, one full-time Protestant chaplain, a part-time Roman Catholic chaplain, a part-time undergraduate psychometrist, and two aftercare/parole officers who were based at Rideau but also served other institutions in the region. There was no organized counseling program with the exception of a community visitors group operated by the chaplain. Occasionally, a specific resident request was handled on a one-to-one basis by whatever professional staff received the request. There was, within the Training Centre, an inmate review board to which all professional staff, correctional officers, and residents contributed. The board evaluated the progress of residents on a regularly scheduled basis.

On the basis of the analysis of resident characteristics and existing institutional resources, it was decided that the major area of need was the development of organized counseling services, which became the focus of the consultant's programming activities. The pattern of high admission rates, short sentences, and variety of needs dictated that counseling services be of the short-term type, structured with reference to specific goals. If a significant proportion of the residents were to come into contact with the program, then group methods appeared most appropriate. Nondirective, open-ended relationship approaches were not entertained on the basis of their apparent inefficiency. Subsequent research and reviews of the counseling literature (Andrews, Note 2) have supported what was essentially a ''judgement call'' at the time.

A package of short-term (1 – 14 sessions) structured group formats, covering a range of specific problem areas, was implemented. The content and the leadership techniques employed were formulated explicitly so that leadership need not be confined to professionals and repetition of the group was possible whenever the number of eligible residents so dictated. Sample areas for specific groups included ''orientation to the rules and regulations of the Centre,'' ''interpersonal skills,'' ''social and moral aspects of the law,'' and ''knowledge of the law.'' A multilevel set of groups intended for alcohol and drug offenders included ''introduction to alcohol and drug use and abuse'' and ''social learning perspective on alcohol and drug use.'' The latter was intended for offenders who recognized a problem with drugs and were making plans for entry into treatment for drug problems. The major counseling methods employed in the groups were the presentation of information in concrete ways, role playing, rehearsal, and differential reinforcement.

The second step was to initiate evaluation of the organized counseling program. On the basis of service priority, methodologic flexibility, and theoretical interest, several of the group formats were selected for systematic evaluation. The research proceeded within a general social learning framework, including a differential exposure and reinforcement model of criminal behavior (Andrews, Brown, & Wormith, 1974; Burgess & Akers, 1966). A series of studies confirmed that under lay leadership structured presentations of information and opportunity for behavioral and symbolic rehearsal were associated with demonstrable changes in various targets including institutional adjustment (Andrews & Young, 1974), self-esteem and interpersonal skills (Daigle-Zinn & Andrews, Note 3), attitudes toward drug use (Andrews, Young, Wormith, & Kennedy, Note 4), and knowledge of the law and legal rights (Wayne, Note 5).

Another major program evaluation was done in the area of citizen volunteers, primarily undergraduate students, as coparticipants in group counseling with the residents. The early history of the community group program has been reviewed elsewhere (Andrews, Brown, and Wormith, 1974). Briefly, an open-ended, nondirective approach to citizen intervention with residents was revised to a format consistent with a general social learning perspective. The focus of the group discussion was narrowed to encompass those specific areas that, while theoretically highly relevant to criminal conduct have been notoriously difficult to manage in routine group counseling with prisoners, i.e., the personal, interpersonal, social, and moral aspects of legal and illegal conduct. Within routine group counseling, residents strongly supported procriminal attitude and value positions. The presence of citizen volunteers, however, introduced variety into the groups, including the exposure of conventional alternatives and more prosocial positions. It was also expected that the presence of volunteers produced a more favorable balance in the patterns of approval and disapproval of prosocial and antisocial positions. Several studies (Andrews, Wormith, Kennedy, & Daigle-Zinn, 1977; Andrews, Young, Wormith, Searle, & Kouri, 1973; Andrews, Wormith, Daigle-Zinn, Kennedy, & Nelson, Note 6; Andrews & Daigle-Zinn, Note 7; Wormith, Note 8; Tully, Note 9) demonstrated that prosocial attitude change occurred when residents were exposed to volunteers, and the amount and direction of change was a function of program factors, volunteer characteristics, resident characteristics, and other types of programs in which a resident was simultaneously participating. As was the case in the counseling studies, the leaders of community groups were most often lay workers, e.g., prison guards, shop instructors, students, and citizen volunteers.

Once the program was effectively underway, the consultants were in a position to draw on the broader community for volunteers and on the Ministry for full-time staff. Within two years the Ministry responded by creating two full-time psychometrist and social service positions and two full-time psychologist positions. The consultant was based at a university where a community-oriented undergraduate program in psychology was developing (Andrews & Gendreau, 1976). Thus the institution had open channels to a substantial pool of enthusiastic volunteers and trainees.

A primary issue in consultation is the maintenance and growth of programs once the consultant exists. It appears that the long-term benefit from the counseling program was the development of a vigorous full-time psychology department at Rideau. The organization of short-term structured groups in the area of alcohol and drugs has developed into a major institutional program. The Alcohol and Drug Program, as it is now known (Kennedy, Note 10), expanded into a joint effort of the psychology, academic, and recreation staff. The latter two departments provide life skills and vocational and recreational training.

In addition, the insistence upon an evaluation component to the counseling program proved valuable in several ways. Psychological staff felt that they were involved in an interesting program, and morale was high. Research grants and contracts made the program economically feasible, and the institutional administrators became increasingly supportive of the department's activities (Gendreau, 1976).

The maintenance of the volunteer program has been another story. At the time of the consultant's exit, the operational responsibility for the volunteer group was taken on by a Ph.D. candidate, and the group continued to operate in an efficient manner (Wormith, Note 8). Responsibility was then transferred to a part-time undergraduate assistant, and the group continued to operate for another year. The maintenance plan, developed by Rideau and the university, provided for continued use of an experienced undergraduate who would be paid to coordinate the volunteer program. It was expected that the student would work approximately eight hours a week and function under the supervision of the university's faculty committee on a criminology and corrections program. The committee failed to hold a meeting for some five months, and for the first time in eight years volunteers were not interacting with Rideau residents. Very recently the volunteer program has been revived again, this time by the Ministry. Rideau has hired a part-time coordinator of volunteers. The volunteers are being recruited at this point on a social-recreational basis, in contrast to a structured counseling format. In one respect this development is disappointing, since research showed that the counseling procedure had the most impact on the residents (see, e.g., Andrews, Wormith, Kennedy, & Daigle-Zinn, 1977).

The failure to utilize the most worthwhile program is in fact all too common in organizations, reminding us of Fairweather, Sanders, Tornatzky's (1974) classic examples of the organizational fact of life that there is little correlation between documentation of program success and organizational commitment to program maintenance.

TOKEN ECONOMY

Since its inception one of the major work programs at Rideau Correctional Centre had been the large mixed farming operation. With changing times the program became less of a viable option. As more inmates were being housed at the institution, management became concerned that there was not enough work available for them. Also, with the increasing numbers more inmates were received who would be classified as behavioral risk problems.

In 1972 the superintendent of Rideau made a specific request of the psychology department to develop a work program that would in part take the place of the now-defunct farm operation. Secondly, the superintendent wanted some of the behavior-risk inmates placed in this program. The psychology department staff felt that a token economy program might be most desirable, particularly in terms of regulating some of the more troublesome inmates. The token economy would be embedded in a vocational and/or industrial workshop. Since none of the current psychology department staff had particular expertise in this area, they recruited a consultant psychologist with the relevant skills.

A number of immediate problems faced the consultant, including a restricted budget for costly material needed in most industrial workshops and a limited range of reinforcers for the token economy. Another problem that arose was that quite a few of the behavior-risk inmates had had several previous incarcerations and were not enamored of the usual mundane work programs to be found in prisons. After exploring several avenues, the consultant suggested a toy workshop to produce items for underprivileged children. The work itself was intrinsically interesting, and the inmates were very much in favor of producing toys for children. These feelings were also reinforced by having inmates themselves distribute the toys to the children in various institutions in the region. The consultant was also able to run the program economically. Most of the material for toys was inexpensive, and the reinforcers chosen, privacy and temporary absences from the institution, did not drain the institution budget.

While the program never gained much acceptance from significant segments of institution administrative and line staff, it did meet most of its goals (Marquis, Gendreau, Cousins, & Wormith, Note 11). A significant number of inmates was employed in the program, and they reduced their incidences of misconduct in the institution. In fact, in one sense the program succeeded too well—the residents' productivity was much greater than expected, with the result that the program encountered space and material shortages. Subsequently the program was terminated primarily because of fiscal restraints. Institution authorities were left with much the same problem they originally had.

The failure of a token economy in a correctional setting is not newsworthy; the correctional literature is replete with such incidences (Ross & McKay, 1976). What is particularly interesting is the fact that the program that eventually replaced the token economy demonstrated that the institution management had somewhere along the way adopted a theoretical rationale for its programming. For example, the work in the counseling area made the point that a differential association model was viable for programming. The token economy produced a group of inmates who had work skills and showed that they could earn and abide by temporary absences from the institution.

What developed was a volunteer program established in settings provided by the Ontario Ministries of Health and of Community and Social Services. In this program inmates worked eight hours a day, five days a week helping the aged and the mentally retarded. In effect, what was created was a differential association model, only applied this time to residents contacting nonoffenders in the nonoffenders' milieu! Clearly, the program was a complementary extension of the earlier volunteer program. From it the program has been expanded, and the outcome data (Gendreau, Hudson, & Marquis, 1976; Gendreau, Burke, & Grant, in press) have been consistent with the types of predictions generated from differential association theory, i.e., residents acquired work-related and interpersonal skills.

IN-HOUSE CONSULTATION

From the brief description provided it can be appreciated that programming at Rideau underwent rapid changes. As the institution adjusted to its new priorities, programming stabilized, departmental programs were integrated (MacDonald, Note 12), and the need for outside consultation lessened. Consultation as a means of problem solving, however, was still appreciated by management. Subsequently, consultant activity was assumed by in-house psychology staff. The psychology department was asked to examine issues crucial to management and line staff. Four recent projects illustrate: (1) an assessment of the contracting of educational services (Marquis & Gendreau, 1975); (2) the organization of staff seminars on working roles and job satisfaction (Marquis & McBride, Note 13); (3) a survey of line staff attitudes towards a proposed program unit; and (4) an evaluation of the effects of disciplinary decisions on residents' behavior.

Perhaps such sensitive issues are better approached by in-house staff and better still when the staff are viewed as not only objective evaluators but also as participants in the correctional environment. It is too soon to comment on the long-term effectiveness of this type of consultation, but it now appears that psychology's value in the eyes of administration and line staff has increased.

Medium and Maximum Security

We have been involved as consultants in seven medium and/or maximum security institutions.

WARKWORTH

Warkworth Penitentiary is a medium security Federal penitentiary located in a rural part of Ontario. It was originally intended to receive residents, many with long sentences, who could benefit particularly from trades training. The institution was built in the 1960s and was expensively appointed with the best in trade program facilities. The impetus for developing consultant services at Warkworth came from the Trent university psychology department, which wished to develop some community liaison. The university is located some 50 miles away from the institution. It was expected that given the isolation of Warkworth from professional services and the fact that many of its residents showed good rehabilitation promise the institution might welcome involvement with the university psychology department. At the time the approach was made (1969) there were some classification services and one psychologist on staff for approximately 250 inmates.

The consultant's initial impressions were that the administration appeared to be progressive and wanted to develop programs. The proposed role of the consultant was to provide counseling services and develop some elementary diagnostics for better classification of inmates into programs. In addition, students would be involved in a practicum where they would provide basic counseling services. The recommendation of the administration to hire the consultant was positive; however, some time later the consultant was informed that regional headquarters had turned down the institution's proposal. No reasons were given for the basis of the decision. Subsequently, the consultant in question became involved in consultant services with an institution from another correctional system.

MILLBROOK CORRECTIONAL CENTRE

Millbrook Correctional Centre is the Ontario Ministry of Correctional Services maximum security institution. It received the most difficult to handle inmates in the Ontario system. Its population consisted mainly of acting-out "psychopathic" individuals, inmates with a history of escape, aggressive homosexuals, residents with minimal intellectual abilities who could not cope with programs elsewhere, and those requiring protective custody. The majority of these residents served sentences of one to two years.

Originally, the institution had adequate professional services, but by 1970 the full-time professional staff had dwindled to one nurse. In addition to the loss of professional staff, security problems were being experienced, and subsequently a new superintendent was appointed to reorganize the institution. In 1970, during this difficult transition period, consultant services were established. The first series of activities were initiated jointly by the consultant and the Planning and Research Branch of the Ontario Ministry. The consultant had been involved in examining the effects of solitary confinement (e.g., Gendreau, Friedman, Wilde, & Scott, 1972) in the Federal penitentiary system. Solitary confinement was used extensively at Millbrook, and the Ontario Ministry felt that an examination of the effects of this type of incarceration was warranted there. The research program was completed (Ecclestone, Gendreau, & Knox, 1974), and the research team gained an intimate knowledge of the workings of the institution as well as the confidence of the new administration. When the new administrator had dealt with some of the pressing security and personnel problems at Millbrook, a second series of consultant activities was initiated. The primary goal of the consultant was to develop diagnostic and classification criteria for resident entry and exit and to establish counseling services. The Ministry cooperated in this venture by hiring two full-time psychometrists, and the consultant involved students from his university. In addition, a social service department was established.

In setting up the diagnostic services, the psychology department routinely evaluated these services and generated considerable information on various resident subsamples (Cubitt & Gendreau, 1972; Gendreau & Gendreau, 1973; Gendreau, Irvine, & Knight, 1973; Gendreau, Wass, Knight, & Irvine, 1976; Gendreau, Wormith, Kennedy, & Wass, 1975; Irvine & Gendreau, 1974; Gendreau & Grant, Note 14).

The Ministry then became interested in aspects of the research and engaged the consultant in a variety of studies centering about the nature and prediction of recidivism (Gendreau, Grant, & Leipciger, 1979; Gendreau & Leipciger, 1978; Gendreau, Leipciger, Grant, & Collins, 1979; Gendreau, Madden, & Leipciger, in press; Madden, Note 15).

After the consultant left for a new appointment, Millbrook authorities continued to augment psychological and social services to the point where the institution now has a viable service program. The only disappointment in the development of these services was that the university did not continue its involvement with the setting, owning in part to the university psychology department's lack of interest in applied work and the consultant's failure, at the time, to establish student involvement in a formal course or practicum framework.

COLLINS BAY AND JOYCEVILLE PENITENTIARIES

These two institutions are Federal penitentiaries handling offenders serving sentences of two years to life. The institutions' populations varied from 300 to 500, and the residents' convictions covered all types of crimes. Those individuals considered to be particularly threatening to internal security were housed at another, nearby penitentiary; nevertheless the security of Collins Bay and Joyceville certainly warranted maximum security designation relative to Provincial standards.

Support for consultant services at these institutions came from the headquarters of the Canadian Penitentiary Service of the Solicitor General of Canada, the staff of which were aware of the consultant's activity within the Ontario Ministry. Following an approach by the consultant, a program similar to that at Rideau was established at these two Federal penitentiaries in 1973. Local institutional authorities were also very receptive to the program. In comparison to other Federal penitentiaries in the area, both Collins Bay and Joyceville had avoided severe internal disturbances. Thus within the context of Federal institutions they were considered stable operations. The programs were run without serious difficulty, although at Collins Bay the local inmate committee was highly politicized, frequently checking the mandate under which the project was operating (e.g., matters of funding, publication rights, project control).

The program (Andrews, Farmer, & Hughes, Note 16) produced results in the direction predicted by differential association theory, although the results were not as striking as those found at Rideau.

Attempts to continue the program failed after the consultants left. Some volunteers tried to reestablish the program but to no avail. The penitentiary service offered to hire the full-time research associate of the demonstration project. If she had entered the service, which she did not, the program might have developed. This experience suggested that program maintenance depends upon the extent to which the institution staff are directly involved in consultant-initiated programs. High involvement occurred at the Millbrook and Rideau settings but not at Collins Bay or Joyceville.

JAILS

The four institutions discussed above are representative of our conventional notions of correctional institutions. The most common institution, however, is the local jail. Most jails in North America are antiquated, inadequate, and bereft of programming (Newman & Price, 1977).

The province of Ontario had been no exception in this regard. Recently the province has attempted to upgrade its jail facilities by creating Regional Detention Centres (RDC). In contrast to the jails, the RDCs usually serve a larger geographic area and have been designed to contemporary correctional standards.

On the surface jails and RDCs may seem to be straightforward institutions in terms of operation and program design, but in fact they are far more complex in many cases than minimum or maximum security long-term holding correctional settings.

Jails and RDCs have extremely high intake rates, and frequently residents are there for only a week or two. Among those who have been convicted of an offence, four distinct classes of residents are found. The first class includes those sentenced on minor charges and fines (e.g., liquor control offenses, breaches of the Highway Traffic Act), sentenced residents who will be forwarded to other holding provincial institutions, those returning for the last couple of weeks of their sentence, and individuals who have been sentenced and are awaiting transfer to a Federal penitentiary.

Of those residents, the ones posing particular problems are those remanded for sentencing or not yet tried (A.R.A. Consultants, Note 17). These residents generally make up 15 to 50 percent of the population. One of the problems with remand cases is that they require a great deal of administrative processing, i.e., frequent court appearances, etc. Some such residents are potentially dangerous, i.e., charged with murder, serious assaults. According to law they cannot be put to work or involved in the usual institution activities. Sentenced prisoners who have been remanded on other charges also prove to be unusually troublesome. They often act destructively to prolong their stay, particularly Federal prisoners who have nothing to lose, facing a return to a maximum security Federal institution. Jail or RDC superintendents are not likely to discipline them, since it will only prolong their stay at the institution, which in the long run causes more management problems. Also, jail/RDC superintendents do not have the option of taking away earned remission, and often they lack segregation facilities.

In addition, some of the RDCs and jails in large urban centers have proved difficult to administer because they have suffered from backlogs of remand cases. By and large, those RDCs and jails in smaller communities, although at times overcrowded, have not felt this problem as much and consequently have posed fewer problems to date for management.

From the consultant's perspective there are several obvious problems. First, the population received at jails and RDCs is extremely heterogeneous not only in terms of social characteristics but also in the types of sentences received and the problems they present to the psychologist. Second, jails and, surprisingly, some of the modern RDCs were built with no space for programs. Third, security is more pronounced than in most maximum security prisons. Fourth, the ethics of dealing with remand cases is complex; in the eyes of the law the remanded individual is still innocent.

Quinte RDC was the first RDC to be constructed by the Ontario Ministry of Correctional Services (1972). It serves a small city and a large rural area. The jail Quinte replaced had always been known to be run efficiently; this tradition has continued since 1972. Quinte had full-time nursing and social services and part-time psychiatric service. The initiative of developing psychology programs was a joint effort of head office, regional administration, and the institution itself. In 1973 a full-time psychologist was hired, reporting to the regional chief psychologist, who was acting as a consultant to the Quinte administration regarding psychological services. Unfortunately, the psychology program did not develop, owing in part to the psychologist's inexperience in corrections and the regional chief psychologist's failure as a consultant to recognize some of the peculiarities of RDCs in regard to programming.

The psychologist left the setting, and it was not until late 1975 that psychological services were reinstituted. Since there was no full-time position available, consultant services were requested. The reporting relationship with the regional psychologist was continued. Two consultants were hired to take over the function of the previous full-time psychologist; both had had considerable experience in correctional settings, which along with the institution's continuing interest in psychological services led to a useful program being expediently established. Four kinds of psychological services were put into effect.

First, the remand cases had to be dealt with. The consultant who became involved in circumstances centering about the client's charges could be subpoenaed by the court. The consultant would be put in the awkward situation of testifying while being employed by the Ministry. Thus the policy developed whereby the consultant counsels the client about problems relating to the client's coping with the immediate environment, i.e., crisis intervention (Kennedy, Wormith, Michaud, Marquis, & Gendreau, 1975). Typically a consultant deals with one to three cases per week, the referrals being self-referrals or made from custodial and social service staff. A second service has been diagnosis and classification recommendations for residents who will be transferred to other provincial institutions.

Many of the offenders coming to the RDC have committed liquor control violations and driving offenses related to the use of alcohol. An alcohol program has been developed whereby five units of material at two hours per unit are presented within a week's period of time. The consultant attempted to match the problem presented by the offender with facilities and individuals in the community who have the services appropriate to the individual.

The fourth program was an assertiveness training program. As a result of a psychometric assessment of the population, the consultant found a group of residents who could be characterized as being unaware of the consequences of their behavior in social situations and of the appropriate responses required. Also, most of the population revealed in questionnaire data a tendency to avoid expressing ideas and feelings in social situations. With this diagnostic information specific goals were set up in the program. The programs were scheduled for two-week periods so as not to suffer from a high dropout rate resulting from the short stays at RDCs.

In developing these programs for the RDC the consultants were very aware of the fact that only limited therapy could be attempted. By at least identifying the problems and making the appropriate referrals prior to release the consultants could start to enable some individuals to make a better community adjustment.

Ottawa-Carleton RDC   In contrast to the Quinte RDC, the Ottawa RDC had been beset with enormous problems since its opening in 1972. It suffered from rapid turnover of superintendents, and there had been numerous escapes, hostage-taking, and internal disturbances. The institution had kept a very high profile with the press and media and had been the subject of several political inquiries.

The first attempt at developing consultant services at the institution failed. Aside from the lack of stability in the institution, the consultant did not commit enough effort to carefully developing consultant activities, particularly programming for the inmates. Also, the counseling orientation (unstructured and nondirective) of staff at the institution was the antithesis of what the consultant felt was appropriate for the type of dangerous offender with which the institution had to cope. It was decided that the best policy would be to wait, and a few months later (in 1975) a second consultant started to cautiously develop services again.

This consultant deliberately played a low-key role, committing a greater period of time to providing services to inmates than the previous consultant and becoming involved in crisis intervention and diagnostics for the consultant psychiatrist. The institution remained in turmoil, and eventually the consultant left to find employment elsewhere. Consultant services were not initiated again for several months, but over this period there was a gradual change in the administration, with a new assistant superintendent being hired who was familiar with psychological programming. Later a new superintendent and deputy superintendent brought stability and direction to the institution. Then two consultants were brought in. At this writing consultant services have developed rapidly. The roles that are carried out are as indicated above, with the addition of assessments and counseling for a developing vocational program. An undergraduate practicum and graduate internship program have also been implemented, with the result that some services can now be covered by the students, leaving the consultants time to assess specific problems and carry out research at the request of the administration.

Brockville Jail is typical of several of the remaining small provincial jails. It serves a small town and the surrounding rural area. Its maximum capacity is 24 residents, and physically it has changed little since it was first constructed in 1842. Typically, programming in jails is even more limited than in RDCs. There are few funds, if any, for the purchase of outside services, nor is there professional complement. A new superintendent appointed to the jail in 1973 had served previously in a treatment-oriented institution in the Ministry. He became aware of consultant services from the Quinte RDC administration and thereupon approached the psychology department at Rideau for services. Because of his very limited budget it was arranged with the Rideau superintendent and the regional director to develop an in-house consultant arrangement.

This relationship with the jail was quickly established, since the administration had a fairly clear idea of the kind of residents who needed referral. It soon became obvious to the consultant that the relationship would be rewarding. The jail was ably administered, and an appropriate rapport had developed between the line staff and the residents. All of the staff were from the local community and frequently knew the offender or his family. They were able to operate very much as paraprofessionals and could advise realistically about prerelease planning with the consultants.

As the program developed, four types of referrals for the consultants became common. First, the jail sometimes receives offenders with lengthy drug histories. These individuals may also be aggressive and act out. For them the jail needed a diagnosis plus an appropriate referral to a hospital upon release. A second common referral is a request to consult with the jail authorities regarding the prerelease plans of one of their residents. These cases usually also involve considerable family counseling, and referrals have to be set up with the appropriate agencies within a community. A third type of referral is that for those individuals who want to remain at the jail, where they benefit from temporary absences and being closer to their families for visits.

A fourth referral is for vocational assessment and in some cases counseling in interpersonal skills. In these cases the jail assigns the resident to Rideau for the assessment, after which the individual is returned to the jail.

Because the reciprocal relationship has worked out, Rideau will on occasion send a behavior-problem inmate to the more secure jail setting. So far, in about half of the cases, the inmate has stabilized and returned to Rideau to complete the program adequately. It is quite likely that the relationship with the jails will continue and be maintained at the current level.

Community Settings

CONTINUING VOLUNTEER CONTACT BUREAU

The overall plan for a comprehensive package of short-term structured groups at Rideau, the center of our initial consulting efforts, included a proposal to conduct prerelease groups, which would link programs and individual resident needs with community services. Left to their own accord, residents oftentimes did not obtain such services, in many instances because they did not know how to find and use these agencies.

The consultant formed a Continuing Volunteer Contact (CVC) bureau in 1973 to meet these goals. Volunteers were recruited and trained to function in an advocate-broker role. The program administration was based at the university. Unfortunately the CVC program faltered because the consultant was unable to develop a continuing financial and administrative base for the bureau. Several methods were tried. A full-time research associate was assigned operational responsibility for CVC on a part-time basis. In fact, the associate's work load was increased to an unbearable level. The Ministry responded by making the bureau the responsibility of a trainee in their correctional administration training program. It soon became clear that a trainee's career interests within the administration program were better served by involvement in Ministry-based settings than by involvement in a university-based program. Responsibility for operations returned to the consultant.

The CVC was subsequently discontinued, since the consultant was unable to place the program within the institutional structure or within the structure of an ongoing community-based agency. If nothing else, the experience helped the consultant come to a personal appreciation of the amount of work required to administer what in effect was a full-time community service bureau.

Finally, it should be noted that even if the CVC had been established adequately it might not have survived. The social services department at Rideau now has developed a viable community-oriented program, and the psychology department followup alcohol and drug program has been improved. These developments do not negate the potential value of a CVC-like program, but clearly some of the roles the CVC program intended to fill have been subsumed by these departments.

ADULT PROBATION AND PAROLE SERVICES

Offenders under the jurisdiction of the Provincial government have probation and parole administered by the Ontário Ministry of Correctional Services. The Ottawa branch of probation and parole had a reputation as a highly professional office. Some of the local administrators had argued for the use of volunteers in probation and parole (Keissling, 1972; 1975) and as a result asked for consultant services, specifically in regard to the design and evaluation of a volunteer probation officer program. The consultant and the agency people produced a proposal; after due consultation with probation and parole staff and local court and Ministry officials, funding was obtained from a variety of sources.

Briefly, the program (Andrews, Farmer, Russell, Grant, & Keissling, 1977) advocated that criminal activity would be deterred if the offenders became involved in interpersonal relationships in which (1) anticriminal attitudes and behaviors were expected and reinforced, (2) social and life skills were acquired, and (3) an increased variety and quality of reinforcement within the community was provided. The volunteer was to function as (1) a model and reinforcer of conventional alternatives and anticriminal attitudes and behaviors, (2) a control agent, and (3) a problem-solver and trainer. The evaluation focused on the specification and measurement of these major dimensions of supervisory process and the identification of the conditions under which supervisory process and outcome were related.

In running the project, the consultant and staff had to deal with frequent personal, interpersonal, and professional pressures; because communication remained open and agency and consultant staff shared common objectives, these pressures did not jeopardize the program (Russell, Andrews, & Kiessling, Note 18). A valuable fund of data has been gathered relating a variety of supervisory process measures to attitude change and most importantly recidivism (Andrews, Kiessling, Russell, & Grant, 1979). In addition, a series of training packages (Andrews & Kiessling, Note 19) on the recruitment, screening, and training of volunteer probation officers has been produced.

The volunteer program is well established and administered by full-time probation and parole staff. The research findings are being translated directly into a new screening and training program for volunteers, and the core materials have resulted in a major change in the roles of selected professional officers.

PRIVATE GROUP HOME AND WORKSHOP

The unit had been a private self-help workshop and group home. The workshop part had existed for five years, the latter for eight. The unit was funded by the Manpower and Solicitor General Ministries of the Federal government. The clients of the agency were primarily young male probationers, parolees, or remand cases.

The agency initiated the contact with the consultant through a recent graduate of the Carleton University–Rideau practicum program. The planning sessions involved both the executive director, who was the "ex-con" founder of the home, and the administrative officer of the home. The goal was to establish a volunteer program, and agreement was reached on supervisory and academic requirements for students. The plan was to begin with a companion-type role for the students and slowly develop roles in the direction of advocate-broker.

Within two months serious and deep divisions became apparent among the administrator, the executive director, other staff, and the clients. The plans of the students, developed with one set of staff, would be ignored or actively impeded by other staff. The consultant's role then became one of surveillance to ensure that the students academic and service goals were being met and of general support and guidance to ensure that the students did not begin to take sides in the internal "battle" and to ensure that students and clients continued to function within program guidelines. Toward these ends, the student-client discussion sessions were moved completely outside the residence setting and held within the university. Under these arrangements the sole responsibility of the agency was to provide transportation to and from the scheduled session.

The program continued on this basis for the contracted period and met with success insofar as the clients were involved in useful community activities. At the end of the academic year (April 1976) the program ended as scheduled but was not reintroduced: in fact, shortly thereafter the majority of the agencies' activities were suspended.

NONMEDICAL DETOXIFICATION UNIT

The detoxification unit for the city of Ottawa is funded by the Ontario Ministry of Health and was established to deal with alcoholics who in the past were dumped into the "drunk tank" and sometimes received short sentences to a Provincial reformatory. The unit was operated by recovered alcoholics and received consultant social services and medical services from a nearby hospital.

The director of the agency approached the consultant with an open-ended request for services and research. Students under the program prepared reports relevant to the agency's interest and students' academic interests. The agency staff contributed to university courses by giving guest lectures and providing on-site supervision. These initial exchanges resulted in a joint proposal to provide a stricter evaluation of the first year of the unit's operation (Wiggens, Collard, Andrews, Hughes, & Loukko, 1976).

The service and research programs were initiated gradually, which was noteworthy because the background situation at the detoxification unit was similar, in several ways, to that of the private group home. In developing the consultation program at the detoxification unit, there was a series of administrative difficulties for the first two years of operation as the staff struggled to develop working relationships among themselves. In contrast to the situation at the group home, the detoxification unit staff and management made no attempt to involve the consultants or their associates in the internal problems; in fact, staff and management at the unit operated to ensure that the consultant process was completed. While close contact with the unit has not been maintained since formal exit, informal reports indicate the unit continues to make use of students and other community resources.

Table 8–1

Consulting Efforts by Conditions of Entry, Participation, and Exit

Consulting Efforts	Entry				
	Institutional Stability				
	Initiation Conditions	Inmate System	Management System	Value Congruence	Knowledge of Setting
Minimum security (RCC)					
Organized counseling	HO, C	Y	N	M	N
Citizen volunteers	A, C	Y	N	M	Y
Token economy	A, C	Y	M	M	Y
Inmate volunteers	A	Y	Y	Y	Y
In-house	A	Y	Y	Y	Y
Medium–maximum security					
Warkworth	C	Y	Y	Y	N
Millbrook—isolation	HO, C	N	N	M	N
Millbrook—diagnostics	A, C	Y	Y	Y	N
CBP/JI—volunteers	A	M	Y	Y	M
Jails					
Quinte RDC I	HO, A, C	Y	Y	N	N
Quinte RDC II	A, C	Y	Y	Y	Y
Ottawa RDC I	HO, C	N	N	N	N
Ottawa RDC II	A, C	N	N	M	M
Ottawa RDC III	A	Y	Y	M	Y
Brockville	A	Y	Y	Y	N
Community based					
CVC	C	Y	NA	NA	N
Probable parole	A	Y	Y	Y	M
Group home	A	M	N	M	N
Detox. center	A	Y	N	Y	N

HO, head office; A, agency; C, consultant. Y, Yes; N, No; M, mixed. AP, action program; AO, advisor/observer. DN, don't know; NA, not applicable.

CONSULTATION ISSUES AND GENERAL PRINCIPLES

To date our consultancy efforts have involved 19 attempts at establishing viable programs. In order to discover relationships among factors crucial to the consultation process and outcome variables, i.e., program maintenance, we categorized the consultation activities on consultation entry, participation, and exit issues (Table 8-1).

Table 8−1 (continued)

	Participation		Exit and Outcome			
Fee for service	Action Program Versus Advisory/Observer	Involvement of Staff in Process at Exit	External Funding Source	Technical Research Reports	Program Maintenance	Influence Other Agencies?
Y	AP	Y	Y	Y	Y	Y
Y	AP	N	Y	Y	M	Y
Y	AP	N	N	Y	M	Y
N	AP	Y	N	Y	Y	Y
N	AP	Y	N	Y	Y	Y
Y	AO	N	N	N	N	N
N	AO	N	Y	Y	N	N
Y	AP	Y	N	Y	Y	DN
N	AP	N	Y	Y	N	Y
Y	AO	N	N	N	N	DN
Y	AP	Y	N	N	Y	DN
Y	AO	Y	N	N	N	DN
Y	AP	N	N	N	N	DN
Y	AP	Y	N	N	Y	DN
N	AP	Y	N	N	Y	DN
N	AP	N	N	N	N	N
N	AP	Y	Y	Y	Y	Y
N	AP	N	N	N	N	N
N	AO	N	Y	Y	M	Y

Entry

INITIATION OF CONTACT

When contact was initiated primarily by the agency or the agency and the consultant, program maintenance was obtained in 7 of 13 cases. When contact was initiated by headquarters and/or the consultant, there was clear program maintenance in only 1 of 6 efforts.

Consistent with Korchin (1976), we found that when the consultation process was initiated by the agency itself the planning and participation phases proceeded relatively smoothly and in most cases agency resources were made readily available. The institution also cooperated in arranging orientation meetings with agency staff, some of whom had taken significant steps in the direction of defining problems that the consultant would have to contend with. Thus we are in opposition to Schein (1969), who argued that agency-initiated contact is not likely to lead to successful consultation, in particular program maintenance.

Our least successful efforts, in terms of program maintenance, were those where the consultant initiated the contact alone or in combination with a directive from above. The failures in these instances were situation specific, and at this time we are not prepared to generalize that these types of contact should be avoided at all costs. For example, the CVC failure was mainly due to errors in judgement of the economic and administrative problems by the consultant. The failure at Warkworth was not due to the local administration. Continuous program development at Collins Bay and Joyceville would have occurred if the research associate of the consultants had accepted the agency's offer of a full-time position to develop volunteer programs.

Finally, it should be emphasized that at the Rideau, Millbrook, Quinte, and Ottawa institutions there was a shift of initiatives from consultant and head office to the local agency. These examples point specifically to Fairweather's (1972) principle of perseverance for successful consultation. With persistent attempts to develop services, these institutions, after initially slow starts, developed and maintained services.

INSTITUTIONAL STABILITY

Unlike mental health, retardation, and many educational settings, institutional stability in corrections generally has two components—the stability of the management system and the stability of the inmate system. Our operational definition of inmate instability applied to those agencies where there was evidence of organized and/or frequent disturbances, i.e., sitdowns, hostage-taking, large-scale vandalism. Management instability was defined as present when there were public displays of discontent within management, management discontent with groups of staff, high staff turnover, and frequent changes in policy and practice.

From Table 8-1 it is clear that institutional stability was strongly correlated with program maintenance. Five consultation efforts were initiated where segments or most of the inmate population were unstable; in none of these were programs maintained. Of eight efforts, there was obvious management unrest in seven; one setting was rated mixed. Program maintenance was achieved in only one of these settings. In nine settings where there were stable management and inmate systems, there were seven instances of program maintenance.

Caplan (1970) expressed the view that institutions with management problems were the most open to consultation. We would argue rather that in corrections, goal-oriented institutions are able to define better their problems, to assess recommended solutions, and to incorporate those recommendations. Two qualifications should be noted regarding the data we have presented. First, a great part of our efforts centered about service delivery to the clients and not reorganization of management or line staff. Furthermore, we would like to think that the increased institutional stability evident at Rideau and the Ottawa RDC were in small part a function of the consultative efforts, which concentrated on delivering a service of benefit to the resident.

Second, our criterion for successful consultation was program maintenance. Consultation efforts described in the literature do not usually employ this strict criterion. It could be debated that a more liberal criterion would be the initiation of a program by the consultant and its subsequent completion with a report provided to the administration as to how to carry on in the future. Using this criterion we achieved some success as consultants with agencies that had had either management or inmate unrest.

VALUE CONGRUENCE

Value congruence is and will become even more of a problem for consultants in corrections. Traditionally, psychologists in applied settings, and particularly in corrections, have been what Szabo (1975) would label as "responsible centrists." Psychologists typically assume the definition of the criminal act as given by society. Delinquent behavior is explained within a normative context. The responsible centrist is an empiricist, operates as if detached from sociocultural and political contexts, and evaluates and develops prevention programs for a goal of immediate social reform.

In contrast, the radical criminology current today is rooted in the civil rights, antiwar, and student movements of the 1960s. Proponents of the view see prisoners as innocent victims of a corrupt state and thus political prisoners (Platt, 1974). Intervention, as psychologists know it, is supposedly a dead end (see Christie, 1970; Martinson, 1975). As a result, ideologic conflicts are common in the criminal justice system (Miller, 1973), and some of these conflicts have affected the functioning of mental health professionals in the field (Silber, 1974). Psychologists committed to the radical criminology position are not common, but in our experience some of the radical criminology attitudes have filtered through to psychology students. Katkin and Sibley (1973) have documented how these kinds of attitudes affected themselves and their students with disastrous consequences. We have also noted some of these values among a few students who have been involved in our consultant work. Our position is that if they view all inmates as political prisoners, they should be encouraged, as Platt (1974) contends, to work outside of the system. If not, then they should be made aware that some efforts within the system can produce beneficial results (Andrews, Note 20; Gendreau & Ross, in press; Palmer, 1975).

A variant of value congruence is seen in how the consultant views existing professional activities in the correctional system. If the psychologists, for example, at the correctional agency were committed to a psychoanalytic model, it would be fruitless to try and develop behavior modification programs.

The data from Table 8-1 indicate that with the exception of two institutions (Quinte and Ottawa RDC) we held values similar to those of at least some of the staff. In the case of Quinte, the consultant not only was unfamiliar with RDC settings, but the staff member who worked on his behalf there became committed to the notion that the majority of clients should not have been incarcerated. In the long run these views made it difficult for him to work effectively, and he resigned. At Ottawa RDC it became apparent early in the consultation phase that there was a serious and in the short term unresolvable clash between the consultant's social learning orientation and selected senior staff's counseling orientation. With no rapprochement possible consultation activities ceased. Later the professionals in question at the RDC sought employment elsewhere, and more fruitful consultation services developed at that setting.

KNOWLEDGE OF SETTINGS

The consultant's knowledge of the specific settings, prior to each effort, was categorized in the following way: Because of our early experiences within the correctional system, we had some minimal knowledge of each setting prior to involvement. Preknowledge was not scored as present unless we had specific information on the program administrative structure and unless we were acquainted with the staff of the agency. Knowledge related to program maintenance. We had thorough knowledge of 6 correctional agencies, and programs were maintained in 4. In 13 cases our knowledge was judged less than thorough, and program maintenance was achieved in only 4 cases.

FEE-FOR-SERVICE

There are three types of consultants, those who are university affiliated, those employed by a government agency who take part in in-house consultation, and those operating in private practice. The authors have most often functioned as ministry-based and university-affiliated consultants; they have not worked as private practice consultants but have supervised the services of other consultants who operated that way.

Table 8-1 indicates that there was no relationship between how the consultant was paid and program maintenance. The successful program maintenance and consultation efforts were evenly distributed under the fee/no fee categorization.

Consultants either operating in-house or affiliated with the university appeared to have distinct advantages in dealing with the consultee. The in-house consultant is well known to the consultees and is familiar with the agency. University-affiliated consultants can draw upon university resources, e.g., student involvement and research, and can use the facilities of the university for workshops and seminars.

Participation

ACTION PROGRAMS VERSUS ADVISORY/OBSERVER
ROLES

Action programs refer to cases where the consultant was involved in designing and operating a program. The advisory/observer role refers to those efforts in which the consultant directed a research program only or discussed problems and concerns with agency representatives. Of 14 action programs, 8 produced program maintenance, 2 had mixed effects, and 4 were failures. As advisors/observers, none of the 5 consultation efforts resulted in clear program maintenance.

These data are relevant to the issue of whether the consultant should "do" something himself or "enable the client to do." Our impression from reading some of the consultation literature is that the two processes are often made out to be distinct, with the latter most often referred to as the appropriate consultant activity. In corrections, at least, the two processes should not be distinct. Moreover, reliance on "enabling others to do" is often too passive. There are occasions when the consultant must provide the leadership, actually run the program, and in some instances ignore the fact that not everyone agrees with given advice and programming.

Repucci et al. (1973) put it aptly in recounting their failure as correctional consultants. As they noted, consistent with their traditional academic training, they were used to "studying" a situation, not "engineering" it. There was a void in leadership at the correctional facility, but they chose to react to events. They found that being skilled observers and interpreters was not enough. Therefore consultants must advocate specific ideas, actions, and values, place themselves on the "firing line," and accept responsibility. In effect they can act as models for efficacious programing. There are solid reasons for adopting this stance, particularly in correctional settings.

Many correctional settings have little in the way of program staff, and competent middle management is still evolving at least to the same extent as in many industrial and educational organizations. Second, correctional managements have traditionally been centralized, and often local authorities are unused to acting on their own. Third, corrections management is constantly preoccupied with crises (Gendreau, 1976) and frequently has little time for program development.

INVOLVEMENT OF STAFF

As noted, the relationship between active consultant involvement and program maintenance was strong. The degree of agency staff involvement in the active program further discriminates between the successful and less successful efforts. The eight successful efforts involved not only active programming but also the agency staff in the programs. The six remaining active efforts did not involve agency staff directly in program roles, and not one of those efforts was successfully maintained. If program maintenance and development is a goal, then it must be planned for. One apparently successful plan is to involve line staff. It is in this sense that ''enabling the other to do'' is a worthy consultant role, but in our experience ''enabling the other to do'' may first involve quite active participation on the part of the consultant and then direct staff involvement.

It is particularly important to have involvement of staff in the program when the consultant is about to exit. We learned this fact to our regret with the community volunteer program at Rideau. Initially, the program had high levels of agency staff involvement. As the university–agency relationship developed and research resources increased, the volunteer program responsibility gradually shifted to the university. This arrangement originally seemed ideal, since agency staff were free to involve themselves in other institutional counseling programs. Unfortunately, such activities ultimately contributed to the collapse of the program. When the university efforts in the program were reduced, the agency staff were committed elsewhere. Eventually this particular consultation effort failed the maintenance criterion.

A final note on the quality of the line staff involvement is in order. In one of the Rideau and Millbrook consultation efforts the consultant's mandates included the recruitment of appropriate agency staff. When these staff arrived the program was enhanced considerably and program maintenance made all that much easier. With the current economic situation the luxury afforded us in this regard is not likely to be replicated. Nevertheless, such situations may occur for other consultants; advantage should be taken of the opportunity.

EXTERNAL FUNDING SOURCES

Consultants, particularly those with research orientations, may bring with them or develop sources of program funds external to the agency. For some time we thought that one aspect of our successful efforts at Rideau was due to the fact that the consultant obtained program funds from elsewhere. Certainly some of the programs could not have been initiated without that support. Review of the data in Table 8-1, however, forced reassessment of our views. Of 6 situations where we received external grants to aid our consultation efforts, in only 1 setting was there program maintenance; 2 settings had mixed results and 3 were outright failures. Consultation efforts with 13 agencies did not receive external funding; 6 achieved program maintenance and 1 produced mixed results.

A partial explanation for this surprising result would appear to rest in the previously noted effect associated with the involvement of line staff and program maintenance. With external funding there was a tendency to rely on extra staff made available via the grants. When funds ran out it was extremely difficult to either hire new staff or reinvolve agency staff in the project. Consultants must reassess the importance that has been placed on short-term, highly-financed demonstration projects.

Exit and Outcome

TECHNICAL RESEARCH REPORTS

As we have noted, the major assumption in our consultation efforts was that the scientist-consultant approach provided a sound basis for consultation. The obvious belief was that consultation efforts would have lasting impact dependent upon the objective reported outcome of the consultant's programs. While we have already demonstrated the number of administrative factors correlated with program maintenance, the data outlined in Table 8-1 demonstrate independence of program maintenance and the production of research reports. That we believed that a positive relationship would exist in the first place is indicative of our naivety. In fact, the lack of any strong relationships between research evidence and policy and program development is not unusual in corrections (Adams, 1974) or mental health systems (Fairweather, et al. 1974).

Some of our early consultation efforts highlighted several of the reasons underlying this funding. Very often we found that agencies viewed research as a luxury and at best a self-serving exercise on the part of the consultants. The antiresearch feeling in some corrections systems has been strong, probably more so than in mental health or educational systems. There are few correctional agencies that have not had unfavorable contacts with researchers. These "ripoffs," as they call them, have been most frequently the result of a student or professor who entered the system, completed a project that was of questionable interest in the first place and of unknown value in the end, and never had the courtesy to supply copies of the project to institutional authorities. Another common problem has been the discomfort produced on site by naive researchers wandering about the correctional institution in wide-eyed amazement at how "normal" the residents are, how stupid the institutional regulations are, or how inhumane is the use of punishment procedures in correctional settings. Of course, at issue were not these facts of institutional life but the fact that the consultant was amazed at finding inconsistencies in the system in the first place. A third and somewhat less frequent complaint is that consultants embarrassed institutional authorities by making public statements that were at best misrepresentative. Finally, a more recent phenomenon that we have encountered is the ''nothing works'' rhetoric (Martinson, 1974) that has influenced some managers and professional personnel in the correctional system. In some cases we have encountered outright hostility and distrust in regard to the experimental method (Hackler, 1974; Matza, 1964).

Our approach to these types of problems has been fivefold. First, we have attempted to document the relevance of the research component as well as modify designs to attend to the staff's primary concerns wherever possible. Second, we directly confront those who espouse the ''nothing works'' philosophy and distrust the experimental method by consistently drawing attention to the many studies documenting reliable and large program effects in the correctional literature (e.g., Andrews, Note 20; Gendreau & Ross, in press). Third, our technical reports now routinely include administrative summaries devoid of the usual technical design and statistical content, and include client and staff evaluations of the programs in addition to the usual objective behavioral indices of program impact. Fourth, we now make more use of oral presentation methods. Where consultant-initiated programs have obvious media impact, we promote this aspect as much as possible. This strategy has worked extremely well in regard to one of our consultation efforts, the Rideau inmate volunteer program. The strong media support for that program has not only enabled the program itself to grow but also had a favorable effect on other treatment programs during times of fiscal restraint. Finally, we include the individual agency staff as coinvestigators, which has been most useful, since word of mouth within an agency is a potent means of communication of program effectiveness.

INFLUENCE ON OTHER AGENCIES

While we were unable to demonstrate a strong relationship between published research emanating from consultant programs and program maintenance at the host agency, such documentation may help to bring about change in other agencies. The last column in Table 8-1 notes those cases where we knew that the host agency effort influenced programs in other agencies. The evidence of influence was citation of published reports by the other agency in their program handbooks or verbal confirmation that staff of the agency were aware of the host agency program and that they introduced components into their own programs. Eight of the ten researched efforts had known impact on agencies other than the host agency.

Research produced by consultation activities also had an influence that could not be accounted for within the limits of Table 8-1. For example, we commented that aspects of the Millbrook diagnostic research were continued and developed by the research branch of the Ontario Ministry of Correctional Services. Recently, leads from that research have been taken up and expanded by the Federal Solicitor General's department. The consultant involved in the original Millbrook consultation has remained involved in a research and advisory capacity throughout. This kind of followup of research by correctional agencies confirms Adams's (1975) findings that corrections agencies are more concerned with and are placing more value on research findings.

Therefore if psychologists are to view their efforts in the broader perspective, perhaps the ''scientist-consultant'' model will prove as powerful in community psychology as some had hoped that the ''scientist-practitioner'' model eventually would in clinical psychology.

CONCLUSIONS

We have reviewed 19 consultation efforts in correctional agencies and related these consultations to issues regarding the condition of the consultants entry, participation, and exit. To our knowledge, this is the first attempt to systematically compare conditions of consultation in relation to outcome across a number of settings. The primary outcome variable was that of program maintenance after the consultants had exited, which was viewed as a profound indicator of organizational change.

Our experiences have reinforced us in the belief that a scientist-consultant model has viability for consultants in corrections. We are also convinced that the utilization of a social learning perspective within this model was a contributor to the success of programs. In contrast to psychoanalytic or group dynamics approaches in corrections, which have produced little in the way of useful programming (Andrews, Note 20), social learning techniques are more amenable to development by consultants with an empirical orientation. With reference to the scientist-consultant model, the research/evaluation component definitely broadened the impact of the consultation programs encompassing agencies and systems other than the host agency, even if the research component did not ensure the maintenance of programs with the host agency.

Organizational impact; as defined by program maintenance, was associated with a number of entry and participation conditions. The reader is of course aware that a number of the consultation conditions covaried. Therefore while we cannot exactly pinpoint cause and effect relationships, we have suggested some basic guidelines for psychological consultation in corrections.

In closing, we wish to make the following points. The consultant who engages simply in sorting out management models runs the risk of forgetting ''who is the client'' (Katkin & Sibley, 1973). At the bureaucratic level the consultant can get lost in the Kafkaesque labyrinth of management games and the resident becomes incidental. At the working level it is often administration personnel who are the "bad guys" thwarting the professional's attempts to help the resident. At the philosophical level it is the entire system itself (Platt, 1974). The facts are that there is no evidence that correctional administrations are inherently more evil than others. Rather, the client will be best protected and served if the psychologist (as consultant) is aware of the unintentional abuses psychologists themselves have heaped on inmates in the name of therapy (e.g., Ross & McKay, 1976). Psychologists are still naive in this regard (Fesbach; 1976, Nassi, 1975; Perlin, 1976) and have been remiss in possibly allowing others (Boyle, 1976; Price, 1974) to take the lead in trying to define the "rights" of inmates and the nature of confidentiality in institutions.

The consultant must be more cognizant of the fact that the process of consultation is a process and phenomenon of interest and value in itself. If we had recognized this fact ourselves we could have systematically collected objective data on the entry and participation phases. As it was we have had to rely on after-the-fact judgments.

Finally, the consultant developing and evaluating programs that focus on reducing the costs of crime and corrections, including means of reducing recidivism among adjudicated offenders, should be aware that the antireductionism and antipositivism rampant in criminology and criminal justice have been associated with weak program designs and even poorer outcomes (Andrews, Note 20). Moreover, the emerging trends toward cost-effectiveness and case-processing models of intervention are vacuous with reference to the identification of program processes and practices associated with positive impact on clients (Gendreau, Madden, & Leipciger, in press). In terms of the available literature the psychologists' knowledge of behavioral influence processes and his research skills are important to the development of corrections. When knowledge and research skills are employed in such a way that agency staff may operate and continue to develop the programs on their own, maximum benefits may be the yield.

REFERENCES

Adams, S. Evaluative research in corrections: Status and prospects. *Federal Probation,* 1974, *38*, 14—20.
Adams, S. Correctional agency perceptions on the usefulness of reseach. *American Journal of Corrections,* 1975, *37*, 24—30.
Andrews, D. A., Brown, G., & Wormith, J. S. The community group: A role for volunteers in group counselling within correctional institutions. In *Proceedings of*

the Canadian Congress of Criminology and Corrections, 1973, Ottawa: Canadian Criminology and Corrections Association, 1974.

Andrews, D. A., Farmer, C., Russell, R. J., Grant, B. A., & Keissling, J. J. The research component of the Ottawa Criminal Court volunteer program: Theoretical rationale, operationalization and evaluation strategy. *Canadian Journal of Criminology & Corrections,* 1977, *19,* 188−133.

Andrews, D. A., & Gandreau, P. Undergraduate training and correctional service. *Professional Psychology,* 1976, *7,* 21−30.

Andrews, D. A., Keissling, J. J., Russell, R. J., & Grant, B. A. *Volunteers and the one-to-one supervision of adult probations.* Toronto: Ontario Ministry of Correctional Services, 1979.

Andrews, D. A., Wormith, J. S., Kennedy, D. J., & Daigle-Zinn, W. J. The attitudinal effects of structured discussions and recreational association between young criminal offenders and undergraduate volunteers. *Journal of Community Psychology,* 1977, *5,* 63−71.

Andrews, D. A., & Young, J. G. Short-term structured group counselling and prison adjustment. *Canadian Journal of Criminology and Corrections,* 1974, *16,* 5−13.

Andrews, D. A., Young, J. G., Wormith, J. S., Searle, C. A., & Kouri, M. The attitudinal effects of group discussions between young criminal offenders and community volunteers. *Journal of Community Psychology,* 1973, *1,* 417−422.

Bandura, A. *Principles of behavior modification.* New York: Holt, Rinehart & Winston, 1969.

Bayer, C. A., & Brodsky, M. J. Prison programming and psychological consultation. *Canadian Journal of Criminology and Corrections,* 1972, *14,* 325−335.

Boyle, C. Confidentiality in correctional institutions. *Canadian Journal of Criminology and Corrections,* 1976, *18,* 26−41.

Brodsky, S. L. (Ed). *Psychologists in the criminal justice system.* Marysville, Ohio: American Association of Correctional Psychologists, 1972.

Burgess, R. L., & Akers, R. L. A differential association-reinforcement theory of criminal behavior. *Social Problems,* 1966, *14,* 128−147.

Caplan, C. Types of mental health consultation. *American Journal of Orthopsychiatry,* 1963, *33,* 470−481.

Caplan, G. *The theory and practice of mental health consultation.* New York: Basic Books, 1970.

Cherniss, G. Preentry issues in consultation. *American Journal of Community Psychology,* 1976, *4,* 13−24.

Christie, N. Comparative criminology. *Canadian Journal of Criminology and Corrections,* 1970, *12,* 40−46.

Cubitt, G., & Gendreau, P. Assessing the diagnostic utility of MMPI & 16PF indices of homosexuality in a prison sample. *Journal of Consulting and Clinical Psychology,* 1972, *39,* 342.

Ecclestone, C. J. E., Gendreau, P., & Knox, C. Solitary confinement of prisoners: An assessment of its effects on inmates and adrenalcortical activity. *Canadian Journal of Behavioral Science,* 1974, *6,* 178−191.

Fairweather, G. W. *Social change: The challenge to survival.* Morristown, N.J.: General Learning Press, 1972.

Fairweather, G. W., Sanders, D. I., & Tornatzky, L. G. *Creating change in mental health organizations.* New York: Pergamon, 1974.

Fenster, C. A., Litwack, T. R., & Symonds, M. The making of a forensic psychologist: Needs and goals for doctoral training. *Professional Psychology,* 1975, *6,* 457–467.

Fesbach, S. The use of behavior modification procedures: A comment on Stolz et al. *American Psychologist,* 1976, *31,* 538–541.

Gendreau, P. Psychological services in corrections: A preliminary report on an empirical model. *Ontario Psychologist,* 1976, *8,* 16–21.

Gendreau, P. Administrative problems and patterns of correctional psychology departments in Canada. *Professional Psychology,* 1979, *10,* 140–147.

Gendreau, P., Burke, D., & Grant, B. A. A second evaluation of the Rideau inmate volunteer program. *Canadian Journal of Criminology,* in press.

Gendreau, P., Freedman, N., Wilda, G. J. S., & Scott, G. Changes in EEG alpha frequency and evoked response latency during solitary confinement, *Journal of Abnormal Psychology,* 1972, *19,* 54–59.

Gendreau, P., & Gendreau, L. P. A theoretical note on personality characteristics of heroin addicts. *Journal of Abnormal Psychology,* 1973, *82,* 139–140.

Gendreau, P., Grant, B. A., & Leipciger, M. Self-esteem incarceration and recidivism. *Criminal Justice and Behavior,* 1979, *6,* 67–75.

Gendreau, P., Hudson, L., & Marquis, H. A. Volunteers in corrections—Why not inmates? *Crime and Justice,* 1976, *4,* 139–146.

Gendreau, P., Irvine, M., & Knight, S. Evaluating response set styles on the MMPI with prisoners: Faking good adjustment and maladjustment. *Canadian Journal of Behavioural Science,* 1973, *5,* 183–193.

Gendreau, P., & Leipciger, M. The development of a recidivism measure and its application in Ontario. *Canadian Journal of Criminology,* 1978, *20,* 3–17.

Gendreau, P., Leipciger, M., Grant, B. A., & Collins, S. Norms and recidivism rates for the MMPI and selected experimental scales on a Canadian delinquent sample. *Canadian Journal of Behavioural Science,* 1979, *11,* 21–31.

Gendreau, P., Madden, P., & Leipciger, M. Norms and recidivism rates for first incarcerates: Implications for correctional programming. *Canadian Journal of Criminology,* in press.

Gendreau, P., & Ross, R. Effective correctional treatment: Bibliotherapy for cynics. *Crime and Delinquency,* in press.

Gendreau, P., Wass, J., Knight, S., & Irvine, M. Psychological services in corrections: The assessment of intellectual abilities. *Canadian Journal of Criminology and Corrections,* 1976, *18,* 190–203.

Gendreau, P., Wormith, S., Kennedy, D. J., & Wass, J. Some norms and validities for the Quick test on correctional samples. *Psychological Reports,* 1975, *37,* 1199–1203.

Gluckstern, N. B., & Packard, R. W. The internal-external change-agent team: Bringing change to a "closed institution." *Journal of Applied Behavioral Science,* 1977, *13,* 41–52.

Gormally, J., & Brodsky, S. L. Utilization and training of psychologists for the criminal justice systems. *American Psychologist,* 1973, *28,* 926–928.

Hackler, J. C. *Why delinquency prevention programs in Canada should not be evaluated*. Edmonton: University of Alberta Press, 1974.

Irvine, M., & Gendreau, P. Detection of the fake "good" and "bad" response on the 16PF in prisoners and college students. *Journal of Consulting and Clinical Psychology*, 1974, *42*, 465–466.

Katkin, G. S. Psychological consultation in a maximum security prison: A case history and some comments. In S. G. Golam & C. Eisdorfer (Eds.), *Handbook of community mental health*. New York: Appleton-Century-Crofts, 1972.

Katkin, E. S., & Sibley, R. E. Psychological consultation at Attica State Prison: Post-hoc reflections on some precursors to disaster. In I. I. Goldenberg (Ed.), *The helping professions in the world of action*. Boston: D. C. Heath, 1973.

Korchin, S. J. *Modern clinical psychology: Principles of intervention in the clinic and community*. New York: Basic Books, 1976.

Keissling, J. J. *The Ottawa juvenile volunteer program*. Ottawa: Information Canada, 1972.

Keissling, J. J. Volunteers in corrections: An ecological model. *Canadian Journal of Criminology and Corrections*, 1975, *17*, 20–34.

Kennedy, D., Wormith, S., Michaud, J., Marquis, H., & Gendreau, P. Crisis intervention in a correctional setting. *Journal of Community Psychology*, 1975, *3*, 93–94.

Lynch, A. Q., & Lombardi, J. S. An experientially based course on consultation. *Professional Psychology*, 1976, *7*, 323–330.

Mannino, F. V. & Shore, M. F. The effects of consultation: A review of empirical studies. *American Journal of Community Psychology*, 1975, *3*, 1–21.

Marquis, H., & Gendreau, P. Short-term educational upgrading on a contractual basis. *Journal of Community Psychology*, 1975, *3*, 94.

Martinson, R. California research at the crossroads. *Journal of Research in Crime and Delinquency*, 1976, *13*, 180–191.

Matza, D. *Delinquency and drift*. New York: John Wiley & Sons, 1964.

McDonough, L. B., & Anderson, T. I. Consultation to courts and corrections. In H. B. Lamb, D. Heath, & J. J. Downing (Eds.), *Handbook of community mental health practice*. San Francisco: Jessey-Boss, 1969.

Miller, W. B. Ideology and criminal justice policy: Some current issues. *Journal of Criminal Law and Criminology*, 1973, *64*, 141–162.

Nassi, A. J. Therapy of the absurd: A study of punishment and treatment in California prisons and the roles of psychiatrists and psychologists. *Corrective and Social Psychiatry and Journal of Behavior Technology, Methods and Therapy*, 1975, *21*, 21–27.

Newman, C. L., & Price, B. B. Jails and services for inmates: A projection on some critical issues. *Criminology*, 1977, *14*, 501–512.

Palmer, T. Martinson revisited. *Journal of Research in Crime and Justice*, 1975, *12*, 133–152.

Perlin, M. On "behavior therapy and civil liberties." *American Psychologist*, 1976, *31*, 534–536.

Platt, T. Prospects for a radical criminology in the United States. *Crime and Social Justice*, 1974, *1*, 2–10.

Price, R. R. Bringing the rule of law to corrections. *Canadian Journal of Criminology and Corrections*, 1974, *16*, 209−255.

Repucci, N. D., Dean, C. W., & Saunders, J. T. Job design variables as change measures in a correctional facility. *American Journal of Community Psychology*, 1975, *4*, 315−325.

Reppuci, N. D., Sarata, B. P., Saunders, J. T., McArthur, A. V., & Michlin, L. M. We bombed in Mountville; Lessons learned in consultation to a correctional facility for adolescent offenders. In I. I. Goldenberg (Ed.), *The helping professions in the world of action*. Boston: D. C. Heath, 1973.

Reppucci, N. D., & Saunders, J. T. Social psychology of behavior modification: Problems of implementation in natural settings. *American Psychologist*, 1974, *29*, 649−660.

Reppucci, N. D., & Saunders, J. T. Innovation and implementation in a state training school for adjudicated delinquents. In R. Nelson & D. Yates (Eds.), *Innovation and implementation in public organizations*. Lexington, Mass.: D. C. Heath, in press.

Ross, R. R., & McKay, N. B. A study of institutional treatment programs. *International Journal of Criminology and Penology*, 1976, *4*, 305−315.

Schein, E. H. *Process consultation: Its role in organizational development*. Reading, Mass.: Addison-Wesley, 1969.

Sebring, R. H., & Duffee, D. Who are the real prisoners? A case of win-lose conflict in a state correctional institution. *Journal of Applied Behavioral Science*, 1977, *13*, 23−40.

Silber, D. E. Controversy concerning the criminal justice system and its implications for the role of mental health workers. *American Psychologist*, 1974, *29*, 239−244.

Speilberger, C. O., Megargee, E. I., & Ingram, G. L. Graduate education. In S. L. Brodsky (Ed.), *Psychologists in the criminal justice system*. Marysville, Ohio: American Association of Correctional Psychologists, 1972.

Stringer, L. A. Consultation: Some expectations, principles, and skills. In P. C. Cook (Ed.), *Community psychology and community mental health*. San Francisco: Holden-Day, 1970.

Szabo, D. Comparative criminology. *Journal of Criminal Law and Criminology*, 1975, *66*, 366−379.

Twain, D., McGee, R., & Bennett, L. A. Functional areas of psychological activity. In S. L. Brodsky (Ed.), *Psychologists in the criminal justice system*. Marysville, Ohio: American Association of Correctional Psychologists, 1972.

Weis, C. M. Evaluation research in the political context. In E. L. Struening & M. Guttentag (Eds.), *Handbook of evaluation research* (Vol. 1). Beverly Hills: Sage, 1975.

Wiggins, T. R. I., Collard, D., Andrews, D. A., Hughes, F., & Loukko, E. *The Ottawa detoxification unit: The first year*. Ottawa: National Health and Welfare, 1976.

REFERENCE NOTES

1. Andrews, D. A. Programme proposal: Short-term structured group counselling. A report to the Ontario Ministry of Correctional Services, August, 1970.
2. Andrews, D. A. Outcome evaluations of group counselling in corrections. Corrections Symposium, presented at the meetings of the Ontario Psychological Association, Ottawa, 1974.
3. Daigle-Zinn, W. J., & Andrews, D. A. Role-playing versus didactic discussion in short-term interpersonal skill training with young incarcerated offenders. A report to the Planning and Research Branch, Ontario Ministry of Correctional Services, Toronto, 1974.
4. Andrews, D. A., Young, J. G., Wormith, J. S., & Kennedy, D. J. The effects of an alcohol and drug information program for young offenders. Unpublished manuscript, 1974. (Available from D.A. Andrews, St. Patrick's College, Carleton University, Ottawa, Canada.)
5. Wayne, D. Short-term structured group counselling and attitudes toward the law. Honors B.A. thesis, Carleton University, Ottawa, Canada, 1972.
6. Andrews, D. A., Wormith, J. S., Daigle-Zinn, W. J., Kennedy, D. J., & Nelson, S. High and low functioning volunteers in group counselling with anxious and nonanxious incarcerated offenders: Effects of interpersonal skills on group process and attitude change. A report to the Planning and Research Branch, Ontario Ministry of Correctional Services, Toronto, 1976.
7. Andrews, D. A., & Daigle-Zinn, W. A structured one-to-one versus group format for volunteers in corrections. Unpublished manuscript, Carleton University, 1976. (Available from D. A. Andrews, St. Patrick's College, Carleton University, Ottawa).
8. Wormith, J. S. Converting prosocial attitude change to behavior change through self-management training. A report to the Planning and Research Branch, Ontario Ministry of Correctional Services, Toronto, 1976.
9. Tully, H. The attitudinal effects of mediated exposure to correctional helpers varying on the indigenous and paid dimensions. Honors B.A. Thesis, Carleton University, Ottawa, Canada, 1977.
10. Kennedy, D. J. The Rideau alcohol program: A multi-disciplinary approach to alcohol related problems of incarcerated offenders. A report to the Planning and Research Branch, Ontario Ministry of Correctional Services, Toronto, 1978.
11. Marquis, H. A., Gendreau, P., Cousins, L., & Wormith, S. Application and social implications of a token economy in an adult institution. In Seminar on Criminal Justice in Canada, Symposium presented at the Canadian Association for the Advancement of Research in Criminology and Criminal Justice, Montreal, 1974.
12. MacDonald, J. R. Assessment of Rideau Correctional Centre. A report to the Superintendent, Rideau Correctional Centre, Burritt's Rapids, Ontario Ministry of Correctional Services, June, 1975.
13. Marquis, H., & McBride, R. Staff development seminar. A report to the Superintendent, Rideau Correctional Centre, Burritt's Rapids, Ontario, August, 1976.
14. Gendreau, P., & Grant, B. A. Predicting assaultive behavior in a correctional

centre, 1979. (Available from P. Gendreau, Rideau C.C., Burritt's Rapids, Ontario.)

15. Madden, P. Factors related to age in first incarcerates. A report to the Planning and Research Branch, Ontario Ministry of Correctional Services, Toronto, 1977.

16. Andrews, D. A., Farmer, C., & Hughes, J. The effects on process and outcome of citizen participation in structured group counselling with incarcerated adult recidivists. A report to the Canadian Penitentiary Service of the Department of the Solicitor General of Canada, Ottawa, October, 1975.

17. ARA Consultants. Prisoners remanded in custody: A preliminary report. A report to the Planning and Research Branch, Ontario Ministry of Correctional Services, Toronto, January, 1977.

18. Russell, R. J., Andrews, D. A., & Keissling, J. J. Some operational aspects of research in probation and parole. A CaVIC module, Ottawa, 1976.

19. Andrews, D. A., & Kiessling, J. J. An introduction to the CaVIC reports. Toronto: Ontario Ministry of Correctional Services, 1978.

20. Andrews, D. R. The friendship model of voluntary action and controlled evaluations of correctional practices: Notes on relationships with behavior theory and criminology. Toronto: Ontario Ministry of Correctional Services, 1978.

Eugenie Walsh Flaherty

9
Evaluation of Consultation

Evaluation is too often viewed by the practicing consultant as superfluous to the primary functions of the consultation process and as requiring knowledge and skills that only the professional evaluator has.

Evaluation as discussed here is of two types, reflecting two aspects common to most consultation programs. The first aspect occurs chronologically prior to actual program implementation in that stage in the consultation process in which the consultant is developing a relationship with the consultee and is planning the specific program to be conducted. In order to plan the program, the consultant must first understand the needs of the consultee. For example, prior to the planning of a training program for social caseworkers in mental health, it would behoove the consultant to have information about the caseworkers' educational background, any prior inservice training in mental illness, the kinds of mental illness occurring most frequently and infrequently in their caseloads, the kinds of clients and problems that the caseworkers feel least capable of handling, any backup supervision available to the caseworkers, and the caseworkers' attitude toward different types and degrees of mental illness. Consideration of such information in program planning will make a program more relevant to the caseworkers and will increase the potential impact of the program on both caseworkers and their clients. The consultant should be equipped with tools and strategies for efficient and tactful performance of this *consultee needs assessment*. The availability of such information can prevent the frequent situation in which a second consultation program with an agency is better than the first because only during the course of the first program did the consultant learn the background and real needs of

213

the participants. Although the collection of this information may lengthen the initial entry stage, the improvement of the first consultation program should facilitate the establishment of a good relationship with the consultee institution and staff.

The second type of evaluation comes into play after the program goals, and the methodology to achieve these goals, have been fully specified. An evaluation approach must then be designed to permit assessment of the degree to which the goals have been achieved. The consultant must design an evaluation approach and select instruments (e.g., questionnaires, existing institutional records, scales, and so on) for an *evaluation of outcome* of the program, allowing assessment of the extent to which each of the program goals was achieved. Given evaluation information of this type, consultants will know the extent to which each of the goals was achieved and can use this information as feedback to improve the consultation program.

In order to conduct effective *consultee needs assessment* and *evaluation of outcome,* the consultant must be knowledgeable about the process required to perform these two types of evaluation, about the instruments and tools available to him, and about the design of administration (or research design) of the instruments necessary to assess *evaluation of outcome.*

PROCESS OF A *CONSULTEE NEEDS ASSESSMENT*

The Behavior Science Corporation (1973) surveyed the mental health consultation services provided by 20 community mental health centers to schools and reported that one of the four characteristics of successful programs was the provision of "services that are relevant to the perceived needs of the school system" (p. 135). Furthermore, the authors found that in successful programs the planning for the consultation often included steps to assess the specific needs of the school for a consultation program.

These successful centers often conduct surveys in conjunction with the schools to determine the needs and interests of school personnel as an aid in planning consultation programs. They then collaborate with the school staff to tailor programs that will be responsive to the concerns identified in the survey. (p. 139)

Thus successful consultation programs are those perceived as providing relevant services and those in which planning includes an assessment of the consultee's needs and interests. It is reasonable to assume that results of the needs assessment, incorporated into consultation program designs, enhance the relevance of the programs.

Montague and Taylor (1971) also cite the importance of program relevance to the effectiveness of the consultation program but stress that the steps necessary to assure program relevance must be carried out *jointly* by the consultant and the consultee:

> Relevance of programs…is a joint responsibility, based on a systematic review of problems, needs, and capabilities. Insofar as mental health workers (the consultants) are the originators and sole (or main) proponents of such study, findings may be imcomplete and weighted with biases peculiar to the particular mental health system. (p. 7)

The findings of several studies that consultants and consultees have very different perceptions of consultation, in terms of the process involved, the objectives, and the roles of the consultant and consultee (Mannino 1969; 1972; Robbins, Spencer, & Frank, 1970), increase the importance of mutual needs assessment as a critical component of joint planning. Such a needs assessment will provide an objective ''foil'' for the preconceptions the consultant and consultee each have about the consultee's needs and interests.

The consultant who accepts the necessity of performing a needs assessment in order to design a relevant program with good probability of success has two major steps to take—the persuasion of the consultee that a needs assessment, jointly planned and carried out, is desirable, and the selection of the method to be used for the needs assessment. The first step will not be discussed here; the situation will vary with different types of consultee institutions, and these have been fully described in previous chapters. However, persuasion of the consultee is only one part of the total process of establishing a relationship with a consultee, a process comprehensively described by Caplan (1970, Chapters 4 and 5).

First Step in a Needs Assessment: Group Discussion

Given that the consultant and consultee have agreed to collaborate on an assessment of the consultee agency's needs, how should they do this?

In planning the strategy, it should be remembered that the needs assessment is often the first contact the consultant has with most of the consultee staff. Staff are frequently administrative personnel and thus not likely to be participating in the actual consultation program. Planning for the needs assessment strategy should thus ensure that the first contact between the consultant and potential consultee participants in the program be one that will enhance the relationship. Common sense dictates that a request by the consultant that the consultees complete a written questionnaire, fill in an attitude scale, or respond to structured interview contacts is not advisable on the consultant's first contact with potential participants. First meetings should include all staff who may eventually participate in the program and should be used by consultants to introduce themselves, or to be introduced by the administrative staff they have had previous contact with, and to discuss the concept and purpose of the needs assessment they and the consultees wish to do. Consultants can then extend invitations to the staff to present orally their feelings about the agency's problems and needs. This discussion should be as open-ended as possible, although it is a good idea for the consultant to prepare beforehand a few questions that might stimulate discussion. Possible examples are as follows:

> If only one change could be made in this institution, what would you like it to be?
>
> If you could have planned your education to train you perfectly for the job you have here, what kinds of courses or practical training do you think would have been most useful?
>
> Of the different clients you deal with, which do you think needs the most assistance? Why?

An open-ended group discussion such as this serves three purposes for the consultant. First, the consultant is introduced to all of the staff, thus facilitating future contacts with individuals. Second, if staff do respond wholeheartedly to the invitation to discuss their perception of needs, the consultant will already be in possession of invaluable information about the needs of the agency. For this purpose it is exceedingly useful to have someone present who can transcribe the discussion verbatim for subsequent perusal, or to tape record the discussion. The consultant should not have to take notes, which will limit participation in discussion and perception of the group's dynamics, such as the emergence of one or more leaders, or of conflicting subgroups among the participants. Third, information is provided that can serve as a basis for subsequent more focused needs assessment. For example, if it becomes apparent that the staff feel that they are getting inadequate support from their supervisors on their cases, the consultant can then design interview questions to assess the specific kinds of cases about which staff feel support is inadequate. In other words, the group discussion can orient the consultant to areas of perceived need, thus allowing followup with specific questions which will provide the detailed information needed to design the program.

Teese and Van Wormer (1975) used a multilevel open-ended discussion approach to assess needs for a consultation program with suburban police. The initial contact was a request directed to a community mental health center for someone to speak to a group of police juvenile specialists and school administrators. Following this presentation, the police officers expressed an interest in learning more about potential applications of mental health techniques to police work. There followed three sets of meetings designed to allow expression of needs and interests by all relevant levels in the police hierarchy. First, the consultants met with a volunteer subcommittee of police. Two immediate needs were identified and the consultants were able to satisfy them shortly. The second set of meetings was designed to obtain administrative support; the consultants met individually with each police chief in the area to discuss their perceptions of needs and to invite them to an organizational meeting, the third meeting in the plan to assess needs. Largely as a result of the individual meetings with the police chiefs (according to the consultants' interpretation), representatives from eight of the ten area police departments attended the organizational meeting to discuss needs and problems. As a result of these needs assessment discussions, the consultants were able to identify four specific problems and to assess subjectively some basic values of the potential consultees; incorporation of such information into the design of the consultation program could be expected to enhance program relevance and effectiveness.

Although the group discussion method is to be recommended as the first step in a needs assessment for most consultation programs, it is rare that information as specific and useful as that obtained by Teese and Van Wormer can be produced by group discussion as the sole method. If group discussions are to be the sole method, it is advisable to hold a series of discussion sessions rather than one, thus allowing the consultant to ask increasingly specific questions as a relationship is established with the consultees. Neff, Lubin, and McConnell (1975) were able to develop a list of eight quite specific goals for the consultation program based upon information about consultee's needs obtained through a series of ''problem-identification'' meetings.

However, as Brown (1967) points out, it is often difficult to obtain specific information on needs in group discussion, and this difficulty may not be alleviated even by holding several discussions:

> The expressed needs of a group in the initial phases of a consultative relationship usually seem to possess a high level of ambiguity, as in ''We need to know more about mental health,'' ''We have a real problem with all these disturbed kids,''...and so on. Needless to say, the expressed needs should be examined closely and given as sharp a focus as possible.'' (pp. 399—400)

Group expressions of need such as those cited by Brown clearly provide insufficient information for program planning; however, they do define for the consultant areas for concentration of attention. What methods can be used to obtain the more specific information about these areas that is needed for planning?

Interviewing for Needs Assessment

There are two methods appropriate to a needs assessment—interviews with consultee individuals in which the consultant has specific areas to explore (determined through group discussion) and examination of existing agency records. These methods are usually the most appropriate at this stage of the consultation process; they will provide valid data and run less risk of offending potential participants, who may be quite critical if asked to complete a questionnaire at this early stage before they experience any benefits from the consultation.

Interviews with consultee individuals offer three important advantages to the consultant genuinely interested in doing a good needs assessment and in building a relationship with the consultee agency and individuals. First, they allow the consultant to explore an area thoroughly; if insufficient information is received from an individual, the consultant may ask again by rephrasing the question or by changing the subject and returning to it later, an advantage lost with a written questionnaire. The second advantage is that if conducted properly, the consultee interviewees will feel comfortable in the interviewing situation, thus enhancing the likelihood of obtaining valid and reliable information; this advantage is also lost in the artificial situation created by a questionnaire. Third, the interviews allow the consultant to develop a good working relationship with consultee individuals by demonstrating concern with their opinions. Teese and Van Wormer (1975) found this a distinct benefit:

> These individual meetings with [police] chiefs seemed to be an effective way of developing administrative support for the consultation program. They still remember that their first contact with mental health consultants was an extension to them, demonstrating a willingness on the part of the mental health consultants to enter the world of the police. (p. 117)

The primary disadvantage of individual interviews is the time required of the consultant. Each interview will take anywhere from 30 minutes to two hours (although the shorter time is preferable) and the consultee individuals' scheduling may not allow more than a few interviews a day. However, the advantages both immediate and in the future (as is so aptly illustrated by Teese and Van Wormer) seem to outweigh the disadvantages. Ultimately, the decision will rest with consultant and consultee. Each consultee agency has unique structures and operating procedures, both formal and informal, that must also be considered in making the decision.

Prior to the individual interviews, the consultee individuals to be interviewed must be selected and the questions must be determined. The selection of interviewees is influenced by the size of the consultee agency, by the hierarchy of staff within the agency, and by the time available to both the consultant and consultee staff. The most important principles to be remembered in the determination of interviewees is that the interviewees should be representative of the consultee staff as a whole and that a sufficiently large number of staff should be interviewed to preclude findings being disproportionately influenced by any particular individual. If an agency or the relevant section of the agency consists of ten or fewer staff, it is advisable to interview all staff members. In the larger agency, the consultant should select at least ten individuals by some method that precludes bias in the choice. It is exceedingly important in the larger agency that there be no bias operating in the selection because the information gained will be used to design a consultation program for all staff, not solely for the staff interviewed. There may be pressure on the consultant to select staff in some other manner, and the consultant must be prepared to present the chosen method's rationale to those doing the pressuring. A common suggestion is that the consultant interview volunteers only. In this case, the consultant must remember that volunteers may have a particular reason for volunteering. For example, volunteers may be a particularly vocal group that will present the agency's needs as more pervasive and critical than they are, an informal subgroup greatly concerned with only one problem area, or staff closest to the administrators who will present an overly optimistic picture.

Frequently consultee agency staff will be organized into formal or informal subgroups, and the consultant may have reason to believe that the subgroups will have differing opinions. In this case, a representative group from *each* subgroup must be interviewed. For example, if a consultation program to a school system is anticipated and there are 5 principals and 100 teachers involved (20 from each school), the consultant should interview all 5 principals and 5−10 teachers from each shool. In the planning for a consultation training program to a security force of 4 supervisors and 40 line staff, the consultant should interview the 4 supervisors and at least 10 of the line staff. Occasionally the staff subgroups will be informal; the consultant must be very perceptive to discern those subgroups not defined in the formal organization and yet representing important factions of differing opinions. Berlin (1973) reports that when a meeting of principals in a suburban school system was held on the extent and kinds of problems resulting from recent changes in the school composition,

> It became evident that there were two major groups of principals: those very concerned with the problems and wanting to alter programs, mostly younger administrators, and those who believed that only a get-tough, kick-them-out-of-school position would be helpful. (p. 35)

In the search for informal subgroups the consultant might look for nonorganizational meetings or activities that formed at the initiative of the consultee staff and that may be relevant to perceived needs. Examples could include a group of teachers who meet on their own once a week to discuss problem children, a group of probation officers who have requested that speakers on mental health be invited, or a group of nurses who have volunteered to spend some of their own time playing with children who are in the hospital for extended periods. Each of these groups will probably perceive the needs differently from the remainder of the staff, and the consultant must be careful to interview a representative sample from staff both within and outside the informal group.

Before conducting the interviews, the consultant should develop a specific list of questions. The first step is the definition of problem areas and of possible causes for these problems identified through the discussions or through other means (including experience with similar agencies). Possibilities for such a list might be low morale (Is it caused by lack of communication between hierarchies? By interstaff conflict?), discipline problems in the classroom (Does this occur with specific types of students? Do the teachers lack perspective and a knowledge of useful techniques?), problems caused by emotionally disturbed children (Do the staff know when a child needs professional help with his emotional problems? Do they know the resources available for this professional help?), lack of confidence in nurses dealing with some patients (Do they lack confidence with all patients or only with specific types? Do they feel most hesitant when confronted with emotional problems that these physically ill patients may have?), and so on. When the problem areas are defined, the consultant should make up specific questions to ask about each one. While the consultant may wish the interview to appear as casual as possible, the casualness should *not* extend to neglecting to prepare questions beforehand. The consultant must remember that while the interview is used to develop a relationship with the consultee individual, it is also used to obtain accurate and precise information about the needs of the agency.

The following is a list of useful recommendations for preparing for the interview:

1. More than one question should be used to explore a given problem area; two or three are preferable. If only one question is used, there is a risk of obtaining little information about the problem because the question is poorly phrased, not clear, or offensive to some of the interviewees. For example, if a potential problem area in a daycare center seems to be child management and attendant discipline difficulties, the consultant might ask the staff three questions: What is the biggest problem when two children are together? What usually happens when two children begin to fight— what do the other children do and what does the person in charge do? What would be the biggest help to you when you are in charge of a group of children?

2 Each question should ask for an answer about a single idea only. For example, the following question is a poor one: How satisfied were you with the consultant's teaching approach and with what you learned from him for use on your job? This question should be rephrased into two questions.

3. The questions should not be phrased in a way that would lead the inter-

viewee to give one answer rather than another. For example, "the consultant helped you to feel more confident in handling classroom problems, didn't he?" or even "Did the consultant help you feel more confident in handling classroom problems?" Instead, try, "Has your confidence in handling classroom problems increased or decreased as a result of the consultation?"

4. The consultant should not use words that an interviewee may not understand, lest the interviewee not want to admit not understanding.

When the consultant is interested in interviewing about the causes of a given problem or in the dimensions relevant in a given problem area, the Critical Incident Technique is quite useful. Basically, this technique consists of asking the interviewee to remember the last time the given problem occurred and then to describe the complete incident. When the consultant has interviewed approximately ten or more people and obtained descriptions of one or more incidents from each, the described incidents can be examined for common elements. If a majority of the incidents contain a common element, the consultant can have some confidence in interpreting this element as an important cause or dimension of the problem area. For example, Spivack and Jamison (1975) interviewed staff of a community mental health center in order to discover the causes of high and low morale at this center. Interviewees were told the following:

We are doing a study to discover the things that happen which affect staff morale. In order to do this we are collecting from staff actual incidents that have occurred recently which have affected their morale. . . . Now, I would appreciate your describing to me something that happened recently that made you feel good or pleased with the fact that you work here. This may include something that happened to you, or to someone else, or something you heard about that helped your morale. (The incident was recorded as given, and then the participant was asked why it affected his morale as it did. After this was recorded, he was asked if there was anything else in the event that made it affect his morale. After this, each participant was asked for a second event that helped his morale, and the same question asked as to why.) Now, tell me something that happened recently that made you feel unhappy or displeased with the fact that you work here, and that hurt your morale? (As with the positive incidents, there followed the standard questions regarding why the event affected the participant's morale, and a second negative incident was elicited.) (pp. 3–4, used with permission.)

The responses of approximately half the respondents were then reviewed for "the essence of the (reported) event which affected morale;" a final list of morale categories, each containing incidents with common elements, was made up and all the responses were scored by two investigators independently. The four largest categories of events affecting morale were support in carrying out job (35%), interpersonal relations on job (17%), inner satisfaction about a job well done (15%), and recognition from others of professional competence (12%).

Caplan (1970) used the Critical Incident Technique to explore the dimensions of helpful and nonhelpful consultations. Nurses who had been involved in a three-year consultation program were asked to describe "an instance in which talking about a case with a consultant added to your understanding or otherwise affected your thinking about the case" and an instance in which talking about a case with a consultant "did *not* contribute to your understanding or your thinking about the case" (p. 314). Caplan's strategy could be easily adopted to explore the dimensions of a problem area involving interpersonal relations in a consultee agency, such as between a principal and teachers, between a supervisor and caseworkers, or between police officers and police chiefs. The most important components of this technique are the following:

1. The question(s) must be very explicit about the problem the interviewer is concerned with. For example, Spivack's questions specifically focus the interviewee on morale on the job, not simply on morale in general.
2. It is best to have the interviewees describe recent incidents; descriptions of incidents occurring more than three weeks before are often less than accurate.
3. As the interviewee describes the incident, the interviewer must write down or record everything said. The consultant who waits until after the interview may forget to include something critical. The use of this technique assumes that the interviewer has little information about the causes of the problem area and therefore does not know what is and is not important. In my experience, most interviewees will feel comfortable with the interviewer writing things down if the interviewer explains at the beginning of the interview that important information may be forgotten without notetaking.
4. After examining the descriptions for common elements, the consultant should ask a second person to independently read the descriptions for the common elements. Only when the two readers agree, by independent review, which descriptions contain which elements can the consultant be sure that the findings are fairly objective.

Additional information on this technique can be found in Flanagan's (1954) excellent article in which he describes background research on the technique, various procedures of administration, analysis of the data, and some of the different purposes for which it has been used.

In any individual interviewing, whether the consultant uses the Critical Incident Technique or not, the following recommendations will ease the process:

1. Before beginning the interview questions, the consultant should explain to

the interviewee the role in the agency of the consultant, the purpose of the interview, and very generally, the topics that will be covered by questions.

2. There is usually no need to identify individuals when performing a needs assessment except by their role (e.g., principals, teachers, counselors). Explaining that the interviewee will not be identified will usually make the interviewee less hesitant about answering questions and hence will supply the interviewer with much more information.

3. Whenever possible, write down the answers immediately.

4. If the interviewee has not answered a question fully, it is best to use neutral phrases to encourage talking, such as, "I see; how do you mean?" or, "Why do you think that is so?" or, "What do you think causes that?" Sometimes a pause by the consultant is helpful; the interviewee may need more time to think about the answer.

5. An interview should be as short as possible, both for the comfort of the interviewee and so that the consultant has more time to interview others. Twenty to thirty minutes is ideal; an hour or more is inadvisable, since interviewees can become fatigued and/or bored.

6. The consultant should practice the interview at least two or three times before conducting a "real" interview in order to be at ease with the process and the questions.

Kahn and Cannell (1957) give a clear and thorough description of the interviewing process, along with several useful sample interviews.

Examination of Existing Agency Records for Needs Assessment

For consultants attempting to do a needs assessment in an agency with which they are not closely associated, existing records are an ideal vehicle for followup on potential problem areas uncovered by group discussion. What is meant by existing records? Bachrach (1972) defines existing records as "routinely recorded statistics [that] are part of the bookkeeping system in use in an institution and [that] are automatically kept up-to-date" (p. 2). Examples of such records are telephone call logs, clinic appointment calendars, referral records, personnel statistics, weekly staff work schedules or logs, case records, memos and letters documenting requests received, achievement tests scores, times between first contact and first appointment, broken appointment records, and patient diagnoses. When considering sources of information for needs assessment, the consultant with an inventive mind should be able to think of many potential sources in the consultee agency's records. An inventive mind, however, is not the only requirement; the consultant must gain access to the records which is not always easy, especially if the consultant has no prior experience with the agency. Brown (1967) points out that ''it should be recognized that agencies, like primitive tribes, have rituals, taboos, sacred documents, and the like, that require special sanctions for the consultant to observe and record'' (pp. 402−403). Regulations governing confidentiality of patient records may also be relevant, and the consultant should be aware of this issue. The possibility of access to records will be enhanced if planning for the needs assessment has been a collaborative effort between the consultant and consultee.

Wingert, Grubbs, Lenoski, and Friedman (1975) describe the examination of health records as an information source for needs assessment on adequacy of health care. They reviewed information on indigent, minority group families visiting large outpatient clinics; the following is a representative sample of the information available to them:

> Forty-one percent of the children and 28 percent of the parents had contacted a private physician for health care in the past. A review of the reasons for contact indicated that the care was largely crisis-oriented and episodic rather than continuous supervision . . . for both children and adults.
> Half of the children had not been completely immunized against one or more specific preventable communicable diseases for which protection is available and should have been provided by that age.
> Of the children appearing in the emergency room, 25 percent had a chronic or recurring illness and the family used emergency room type of intermittent crisis-oriented care as the sole approach to medical care.
> Compliance in keeping scheduled appointments was only 52 percent in specialty clinics. (p. 850)*

They concluded that the information provided by the records indicated that these families required assistance in order to receive adequate health care, that the present staff of doctors and nurses could not provide the kind of assistance needed, and that a possible solution would be the addition of ''the indigenous, trained health aide, who shares common ethnic origin, language, and group interest.'' A program was then planned for the health aides in which they would provide comprehensive health care supervision and coordination for the indigent families in a manner that the authors hoped would improve some of the conditions uncovered in the needs assessment.

Lane and Kelman (1975) have compiled an exhaustive list of indicators of physical and psychological maternal health care quality, many of which can be obtained from records maintained on ambulatory and hospital records. For example, indicators of accessibility (a criterion of importance in most service delivery systems) available from existing records are patient occupational and educational data and methods of payment and prepayment. These indicators

*From Wingert, W.A., Grubbs, J., Lenoski, E.F., & Friedman, D.B. Effectiveness and efficiency of indigenous health aides in a pediatric outpatient department. *American Journal of Public Health*, 1975, *65*, 849−857. Used with permission.

could provide an assessment of an institution's service accessibility to low-income families. Indices of the effectiveness of the care delivered that are available from records are broken appointments, maternal and infant mortality or complications, prematurity, extended length of stay, and use of family planning (post partum). These indices might pinpoint areas of care in need of improvement.

Examination of personnel records may also uncover problem areas. Staff logs provide a wealth of data on broken and canceled appointments, on time spent on particular kinds of activities such as direct client care, maintenance of patient records, and home visits, and on the relationship of time spent in supervision to time spent in providing care. Such data may indicate a need for a new system of patient followup, for a simpler patient record system, for inservice training in maintaining records efficiently or in home visit strategies, or for a change in method of supervision [see St. Clair, Silver, and Spivack (1975) for more suggestions on the use of staff log information]. Examination of the minutes of staff meetings over a period of time may indicate a particular problem area that is never completely resolved and thus reappears periodically. Referral records may reveal overutilization of some community resources and underutilization of others or referral of particular types of clients only. Examination of telephone logs may provide indications of the adequacy of the present crisis intervention system.

Although the needs assessment approaches described here are those that will usually be most convenient and effective for the consultant, there are many other strategies for needs assessment [see especially Warheit, Bell, and Schwab (1974) and Hargreaves, Attkisson, Siegel, McIntyre, and Sorensen (1974)].

ASSESSMENT OF INDIVIDUAL PARTICIPANTS' NEEDS

When the needs assessment has achieved its goal of delineating the needs of the consultee agency and of its staff, the consultant and consultee have two tasks: first, to decide together what they think objectives or goals of the consultation program should be, and, second, to design the program itself (the curriculum, the schedule, the participants, and so on). Miller (1975), relevant to the first task, discusses thoroughly the objectives in continuing education programs. The second task is dependent for the quality of its results on the depth of the needs assessment, on the collaboration of the consultant and the consultee, on the participation of relevant consultee staff in the plans (including representation of those who will be involved in the actual program), and on the experience and training of the consultant. The experienced consultant will know that the best program design requires not only the results of the needs assessment but also certain information about the background and needs of individual participants. It is especially important in the design of staff development consultation programs that the consultant know the educational and employment background of the participants as well as any other previous exposure they may have had of relevance to the planned program. Guttentag, Kiresuk, Oglesby, and Cahn (1975) emphasize the necessity of such information for an effective program:

> In planning programs, the use of information about the needs of individual trainees varies with respect to the type of program. . . . In continuing education programs individual trainee needs should be taken into account when planning programs. In in-service programs, where emphasis is on the specific practice of specific individuals, individual trainee needs should be sampled in detail and should be directly used in the planning of the program. In general, the more factual and complete the information about the trainee needs, the better the program. (p. 44)*

Such information can be critical to the success of the program as designed. For example, in planning a consultation program to a hotline for child-abuse, as a consultant, I found two data about the participants critical to program success. First, all of the hotline staff had received inservice training in Rogerian, reflective listening techniques. While the consultants personally disagreed with the efficacy of the approach as the sole technique, they felt that in this first consultation effort with this agency it was important not to present alternate listening techniques. Such training would have presented two potential problems, conflict with the hotline agency that sponsored the inservice training and an unfair disadvantage to the staff, who would then have to decide individually on the technique they favored. Therefore the consultants designed the program curriculum to supply a known need of the staff, lack of knowledge about child development, and carefully avoided discussion of listening techniques except in answer to questions. The consultants also found, through assessment of the individual participants' needs, that virtually all of the hotline staff were volunteers. This meant that scheduling must be suited closely to their convenience, or there was a real risk of low attendance. The program was therefore held in the evenings in a few long sessions instead of in more frequent short sessions. All involved agreed after program termination that any other plan would have resulted in minimal attendance.

Collection of information about participants' educational and employment background can sometimes be obtained through records maintained by the agency. If these are incomplete or unavailable, the consultant can design a brief written form for the potential participants to complete, explaining to them that the information is needed for design of a program suited to their needs and nonredundant with their previous experience. This form should also request information on the participants' scheduling desires, topics they especially wish to see included (the consultant might include a list derived from

---

*From Guttentag, M., Kiresuk, T., Oglesby, M., & Cahn, J. *The evaluation of training in mental health*. New York: Behavioral Publications, 1975. Used with permission.

the previous needs assessment), and the participants' expectations of the program. Cutler and McNeil (1966) describe a Personal Data Sheet designed to collect such information from teachers in a school mental health consultation program and present an analysis of the relationship of this information to extent of program participation; knowledge of such relationships could be very useful to the consultant in the planning of subsequent programs.

PROCESS OF *EVALUATION OF OUTCOME*

Needs of the consultee agency and participant staff have been assessed, objectives have been defined, and a program has been designed to achieve these objectives; now the consultation program is ready to begin right? Wrong: how are the consultee and consultant going to know if the objectives have been achieved? They can reply, as have so many in the past, on subjective impressions but they are probably experienced enough to distrust such impressions as the *sole* source of feedback. Such impressions have their place in conjunction with more objective information. The methods I describe are those that can be carried out by a consultant without professional expertise in evaluation.

Evaluation by Means of Simulated Situations

One of the ultimate objectives of most consultation programs is to effect behavioral change in the consultee participant's attitude toward some concept or in the participant's self-esteem; however, it is generally accurate to say that the consultant hopes that the attitudinal or self-esteem questions will be a stepping stone toward a behavioral change. This situation poses a problem for evaluation. The most accurate and direct method of assessing behavioral change would be to observe the participant's behavior in some relevant situation before the consultation program, to observe it again after program termination, and to describe in some manner the important changes. Logistically this method of evaluation is difficult even for an in-house evaluator; it is usually impossible for an out-of-house consultant. In order to observe the participant in the relevant situation, the consultant might have to follow him about at work all day; few participants would agree to this, and few consultants have the time. Consultation to teachers in a school setting is sometimes an exception to this logistical problem, since teachers are usually a "captive audience" in the classroom much of the day and are interacting with the students most of this time.

The consultant has an alternative to following the participant about, hoping that the relevant situation will come up. The consultant can create a "simulated situation," identical to the actual job-related situation that is of interest, and have the participant role-play. By observing role-playing before and after the consultation program, the consultant can observe change (or lack of change) in the behavioral dimensions deemed important to the program's objectives. This method is particularly effective in the evaluation of a consultation training program for staff in a hotline or crisis telephone capacity, as France (1975) comments:

> Simulated calls seem to provide the best opportunity for systematically evaluating how well volunteers perform the behaviors expected of them. Well-trained role players cannot be distinguished from actual callers…, yet the experimenter retains control over the type of situation the worker is required to deal with. (p. 214)

In my experience, however, even simulated situations in which the participant role-plays (or is led to believe that the situation is genuine, as France suggests), are logistically unwieldy. Time must be arranged before and after the actual program for the consultant to observe each participant role-play individually. In addition, a third party must contribute time by playing a role (such as the telephone caller). Furthermore, the consultee participant who is role-playing while being observed cannot help but feel self-conscious, which may result in unnatural behavior yielding unreliable and possibly invalid data.

The consultant can avoid these difficulties and still evaluate by means of a simulated situation, by describing the simulated situation on paper and asking participants to provide written descriptions of their responses to the situation. Clearly these responses will not be identical to those in the genuine situation. The most obvious difference is that participants will describe only portions of their responses because it takes more time to write descriptions of responses than to actually perform them.

Given that the consultant can expect to read a limited description, the simulated situation must be so structured that the participant describes those responses relevant to the program's goals and not just any responses occurring in the situation. For example, I created several simulated situations for the evaluation of a consultation program for nurses on maternity and pediatrics wards. One objective of the program was to heighten the nurses' awareness of the importance of the emotional interaction between mother and child as a source for the child's apparently physical problem. Two of the simulated situations were described as follows:

1. Suppose that when a mother held her newborn baby, the baby was rigid and unresponsive.
2. Suppose that you are working with a teenage mother and her first baby.

The nurse was then asked to answer two questions:

1. What are the things, if any, you as the attending nurse would do?
2. What are the three *questions*, if any, you would ask?

Note that these questions were designed to evoke responses relevant to the objective described above by eliciting a description of actions and questions that should reflect the nurses' orientation. The nurses completed the questionnaires in the beginning of the first program session and in the last session and examination of the responses revealed a shift from attribution of the child's problems to physical causes toward increasing awareness of the mother-child emotional interaction.

Caplan (1970) used the simulated situation method to evaluate a three-year consultation program for public health nurses. A fictitious case record was made up involving two families presenting a large variety of health-related problems, and the nurses were asked to respond to two questions about the case: "What are some of the important problems in this situation?" and, "What, if anything, do you think a nurse could do in this situation?" (p. 316). After they responded in writing, the nurses were interviewed about their responses; these interviews, although helpful in interpretation of the responses, could be omitted by the time-limited consultant. The nurses' responses were rated for "objectivity."

Simulated situations have also been used for the evaluation of consultation to school staff. Keutzer, Fosmire, Diller, and Smith (1971) describe the evaluation of a two-week consultation program for the staff of a new high school in which the objective was to facilitate an effective social system among the staff. One of the evaluation instruments was the 25-item Situation Prediction Questionnaire (SPQ), in which the participants were asked to predict their own behavior in five types of social interaction that could be expected to occur frequently among the staff. The participants complete the SPQ before and after the program and at later times through the school year.

Cutler and McNeil (1966) used a questionnaire that tapped how teachers handled serious classroom problems in their evaluation of an extensive consultation program to teachers; the teachers completed this at the beginning and end of the program.

The consultant who wishes to use the simulated situation method must be very careful in designing the procedure to assure useful information. The following suggestions are generally helpful:

1. The behaviors that the program is designed to change must be described concretely so that there can be no doubt about whether a given behavior is or is not relevant. The description of the behavior should be a joint product of the consultant and the consultee.

2. Next, several situations must be selected in which the relevant behaviors are most likely to occur. These situations should be fairly common to the participants' working situation. In my experience the participants themselves are the best source of what constitutes a common and relevant situation. The consultant, after describing the situations, should ask consultee staff who will not be involved in the program itself to read the

descriptions for accuracy and comprehensiveness; the descriptions must fully convey the situations. It is best to employ at least two (or better, three) situations to assure that at least one will be common for each participant. Occasionally, too, a situation does not elicit many responses for reasons that the consultant did not forsee.

3. One or more questions should be made up that the participants will answer for each situation. The questions should be worded to obtain descriptions of the relevant behaviors from the participants [see my description of the program for nurses as well as Caplan's (1970), above].

4. The participants should complete the questionnaires before the training program actually begins and after it ends. It is important to provide them with ample time to think and write.

5. To score the responses, it is best to begin with a sample of the responses from each of the two testing periods. One rater should read them and categorize the behaviors as he or she deems appropriate. Classifications could be made by type of response ("ignores client's question" and "suggests possible solution to client's problem"), by degree of desirability of response ("very helpful," "moderately helpful," "slightly helpful," and "not at all helpful"), and by extent ("offers three alternative solutions," "offers two…" and so on).

6. The first rater, when satisfied with the scoring, should ask a second rater to score the responses, giving that rater the scoring system but not the specific scores. Any differences in scoring of specific responses should be discussed and resolved to mutual agreement.

7. When the two scorers have independently scored all responses and found agreement on the scoring of most responses (90 percent is a good standard to set), the consultant can be satisfied with the scoring and begin to compare the scores from before and after the program.

Morgan and King (1975) describe a more structured simulated situation method developed by trainers at the Roadhouse, Colorado State University's crisis center (Delworth, Rudow, & Taub, 1972) that can be used for the evaluation of telephone counselors' discrimination ability concerning responses to callers' problems. Telephone counselors are presented with the Crisis Center Discrimination Index (CCDI), consisting of 16 representative excerpts of calls to a crisis center. Four hypothetical responses follow each excerpt, and the participant rates each hypothetical response on a scale of 1 to 5 (5, most helpful). The excerpts present a variety of problems designed to be representative of typical telephone calls received at a crisis center. The participants' answers are structured by having them rate the helpfulness of each hypothetical response. The hypothetical responses have also been rated independently by the CCDIs authors, and the difference between the authors' overall score and the individual participant's score is said to reflect the participant's discrimination ability.

This general approach lends itself to adaptation in a variety of evaluation situations. For example, in a consultation training program for caseworkers that has the objective of improving the caseworkers' interviewing techniques, the consultant could devise several simulated situations in which a client presents a caseworker with a problem; a variety of hypothetical responses would be provided that would be rated independently by several experienced caseworkers along dimensions deemed relevant to the program's objectives (supportiveness, degree to which question will elicit necessary information, specificity and appropriateness of solutions offered, and so on) and an average of the experienced caseworkers' ratings obtained for each hypothetical response. The program participants would then complete the questionnaire before and after the training program.

A similar approach could be used to evaluate the helpfulness of school counselors' responses to a troubled child or parent, the supportiveness of a worker in a geriatric facility to a senile patient disturbed about something, or any other situation in which the consultation program participants are being trained in responding to a problem situation.

Evaluation by Means of Supervisor and Peer Ratings

The discussion of the simulated situation method began with the assumption that behavioral change is the final objective of most consultation programs and that observation by the consultant of the participants at work, as a means of assessing behavioral change, was usually logistically impossible. However, the consultant may be able to enlist the assistance of those who would be observing the participants at work anyway—supervisor and peers. If the supervisor or peers can objectively rate the participants' behavior in the relevant situation, they will provide the consultant with ratings based on extended observation and actual experience.

Morgan and King (1975) have developed a 12-item rating scale, the Telephone Counseling Effectiveness Scale (TCES), to be used by a rater assessing a telephone counselor on the dimensions of "accurate empathy, nonpossessive warmth, and genuineness" (p. 243). Each of the three dimensions is represented by four specific verbal behaviors, and the rater scores the frequency with which the telephone counselor exhibits each of the 12 behaviors in answer to a telephone call (e.g., never, almost never, sometimes, often, almost always, and always). Morgan and King used simulated telephone calls and the participants were informed that the calls were simulated; however, the rating scale would be quite appropriate for use by a supervisor or peer observing a participant answering genuine calls. Neff et al. (1975) had co-workers (subordinates, peers, and superiors) of police participating in a training program rate the participants' behavior at various points during the program. Four dimensions of behavior were tapped in a 26-item questionnaire; for example, the behavior dimension of "communication" might be partially assessed by an item reading, "In the area of communication, is the subject understood by others?" The co-workers rated the participants on each item along a seven-point scale from "rarely" to "almost always."

Supervisor and peer ratings as an evaluation method may appear deceptively simple, but there are certain steps that must be followed or the information produced will be of little value:

1. The attributes for the ratings should be directly related to the objectives of the program and should be agreed upon by both the consultant and the consultee involved in planning.

2. The attributes that the participants will be rated on must be defined as concretely as possible. For example, instead of asking for rating on "ability to communicate with people," the consultant should select several specific behaviors that reflect an ability to communicate, such as "the subject's instructions are clear and easily understood," or, "when someone tells the subject about a problem, the subject's comments show he or she was really listening to them," etc. The consultees should examine the behaviors to make sure they are relevant to the work situation of the participants.

3. Every behavior to be rated should be followed by a scale of frequency with four to seven points. The number of points on the scale will depend upon the extent to which the consultant and consultee think the rater can discriminate the specific behavior.

4. The rater should preferably not be aware of the objectives or specific content of the consultation program; this may influence the ratings.

5. More than one rater should be used if at all possible in order to avoid possible biases of a single rater.

6. If possible, the rater should also rate people who are not participating in the program and should not know which persons are in the program.

7. The ratings should be carried out before the consultation program begins and again after it ends. Ideally, the rater should have forgotten the first set of ratings when doing the second set. In any case, the consultant should not let the rater see the original ratings, taking them as soon as they are done.

Evaluation by Means of Existing Agency Records

Existing records are also useful for evaluation of program outcome. The variety of records described earlier opens up many potential sources of information for assessing change brought about as a result of consultation. As stated earlier, the consultant with an inventive mind should be able to translate many of the program's objectives into information available on records already maintained. The advantages of using existing records for evaluation have been fully described by Webb, Campbell, Schwartz, and Sechrest (1966) in their chapters on archival records. The primary advantage is that existing records are an "unobtrusive" evaluation technique in that the program participants are not aware that they are being evaluated, as they are when completing a questionnaire or answering interview questions. This "unobtrusiveness" enhances the probability that the consultant is obtaining valid information about behavioral change.

There is an additional advantage specifically for the consultant doing evaluation. The consultant is dependent upon the permission and cooperation of the consultee agency staff in a way that the in-house evaluator is not and must obtain permission for any evaluation instrument; this permission may be difficult to obtain when the staff are suspicious of "being tested," a problem I have encountered frequently. If permission is given, the evaluator must depend on the cooperation of the agency staff to complete written forms and keep appointments for interviews or observations. Even when staff are cooperative, scheduling problems, over which the out-of-house consultant has little control, may intervene. Frequently the consultant will have data on some participants from before but not after the program. When using existing agency records, the consultant avoids these problems (although others may be encountered; see below) and can anticipate obtaining valid information.

What kinds of records will reflect the behavior specified in the objectives of the program? This question can best be answered by describing the uses to which records have been put in the evaluation of a variety of programs. Stephenson (1973) used information from a variety of records to demonstrate the effect of four years of mental health consultation by a consultant from the psychiatry department of a university to a child and family welfare agency. The consultation was typical of many long-term consultation programs in that it involved a variety of types of consultation—direct and indirect consultation, staff training, and a joint research demonstration project. The objectives of such a multipronged program are difficult to define specifically, but there are several changes, reflected in existing records, that are reasonable to accept as indicative of success or failure of the consultation program. Referral records were examined for a change in the percentage of cases referred to an outside psychiatrist. Attendance of children from the agency at the local emergency department was compared to attendance from another child welfare agency in the city that did not have a psychiatric consultant. Requests from the agency for the different types of consultation were tracked, as well as the time spent by the consultant on the various types, to see if the number and kind of requests changed. Records of the ages of the children referred were examined; the average age decreased over the four years, suggesting "earlier identification of problems and more awareness of the significance of the effect of early experiences" (p. 258). It is worthwhile to read Stephenson's interpretation of the findings from the various records, since she recognizes the caution one must take in inferring the behavioral and attitudinal changes that led to the findings on the records.

Wingert, Grubbs, Lenoski, and Friedman (1975) also used a variety of existing records to evaluate the effectiveness of placing indigenous health aides in a pediatric outpatient department. The objective was to improve the health and social welfare of indigent families by increasing followup and coordination to these families through the aides. After one year the performance of the aides was compared to the performance of public health nurses (PHNs) by means of several routine records. The health and social surveys to be done for each family were compared for percentage of total items (2205 items) completed. The ability to identify problems and the ability to correct identified problems (pediatric and adult independently) was compared by examination of records maintained by the PHNs and aides on the family's health and social progress. An important objective of the program was to increase the percentage of scheduled appointments kept by the families; the progress records were checked for number and type of appointments kept. The progress records were also checked for change in a variety of social variables obtained by the family during the year, such as welfare, food stamps, adequate clothing, and so on. Note that although the authors did not contact the families directly to interview them for information, comprehensive and probably quite accurate data about changes in the families' health and social status were obtained from routinely maintained records. No additional data collection was required for this thorough evaluation.

Dorsey, Matsunaga, and Bauman (1964) used regularly maintained referral forms as one means of evaluation of a five-month mental health consultation program for public health nurses and found that there was an increase of referrals of clients who were "exposed to potential mental health hazards and situations"; the nurses seemed to be placing more emphasis on prevention. Three changes were found in the information recorded on the referral forms: an increase in data on the clients' "total functioning in daily experiences," an increase in information recorded about the clients' background, and an increase in information about the clients' fathers. The authors reported detailed findings on 18 types of information that might be recorded on a referral form for the first two cases, middle two cases, and last two cases for each nurse.

Attendance records are a very satisfactory method of doing a preliminary evaluation, and the data are usually readily available on agency records. Krebs (1971) admits that attendance is a "global measure" in that there are many reasons why someone may or may not attend an event. However, he argues that attendance has face validity as a gross indicator of people's motivation:

It seems reasonable to assume that basically a person attends a program because it is seen by him or her as worth the effort involved to attend. Most program directors are probably already using attendance as a basic indicator of the success of their program. If no one comes, the program has obviously failed; if people come, the possibility exists that they have been helped. (p. 73)*

Krebs used attendance to evaluate the effectiveness of community workers in getting patients to keep appointments for followup care after discharge from a state hospital. Records of attendance at the initial followup visit were used, and a positive relationship was found between the hiring of the community workers and attendance.

Wingert et al. (1975) used appointments kept and broken by clients to evaluate their similar program. Stephenson (1973) reports on the attendance of children from the consultee agency at a local emergency department as a measure of evaluation.

The experience of Tobiessen and Shai (1971) with attendance figures illustrates the care one must use in interpretation. In comparing individual and group mental health consultation with teachers, they found that attendance was very poor for two of the four groups. High attendance at the other two groups was attributed to "very active principal involvement" in one group and "compulsory attendance in order to receive inservice credit" in the second (p. 220). Attendance was an ideal means of evaluating the effect of these two motivating forces because it seemed to reflect their presence very closely. There are a variety of sources in which attendance information may be available, including patient records, referral records, activity logs maintained by staff, and sign-in sheets for group meetings.

Staff time utilization records, or staff activity logs, can provide a wealth of information for evaluation. Most agencies maintaining logs do so for payroll information, for client billing, for supervision, and occasionally to track staff activities. If maintained for payroll or client billing purposes, the records will probably be up-to-date and fairly accurate. Data on such records are especially useful for evaluation of program consultation. For example, if institutional changes are recommended to increase efficiency, data on the logs before and after the changes are made can be compared. Program changes designed to improve morale can be evaluated by looking at sick-time, check-

---

*From Krebs, R. Using attendance as a means of evaluating community mental programs. *Community Mental Health Journal*, 1971, 7, 72–77. Used with permission.

in-time, number of cases or clients seen, and so on; changes made with the purpose of improving efficiency may be reflected in time spent on particular activities, time spent between activities, numbers of cases seen or products completed, and so on. St. Clair et al. (1975) describe the use of log information to assess the effect of administrative measures designed to increase the amount of time spent with clients. Flaherty and Martin (1976) used log information to examine the results of program development and specific administrative decisions.

This discussion of the utility of existing records as a means of evaluation has by no means mentioned all the possible sources; the available sources will vary with the size and especially with the type of agency. Webb et al. (1966) discuss evaluation with actuarial records (records of birth, marriage, divorce, death), the Congressional Record (one might examine the minutes of meetings in any institution), personnel records, judicial data, budget data, sales records, accident records, and productivity or output records, to mention those of greatest potential use to consultants.

Using existing records for evaluation is not problem-free, however. The discussion by Webb et al. (1966) of the difficulties involved with these records is entertaining and thorough, and Bachrach (1972) describes a case study of the use of referral forms and the difficulties one should anticipate. Some of the more frequent problems are as follows:

1. *Missing information,* which can be in the form of missing records or of records with unrecorded items. The consultant using incomplete records should try to find out if the losses are random or selective (e.g., cases reflecting poorly on someone's performance may never have been recorded, records from one particular unit may be lost, and so on).
2. *Illegible or incomprehensible information.* The consultant may be able to enlist the aid of agency staff in interpretation.
3. *The recording system,* or the components that the consultant needs, may have been instituted too late for baseline data prior to consultation, or may not be used by all agency staff (the latter problem is especially likely in the case of staff utilization records).

Sometimes the problems can be compensated for or are of insufficient magnitude for the consultant to reject the use of such records. Existing records can be so fruitful in terms of evaluating information that every consultant should examine all possibilities among the consultee agency's records.

Evaluation of Attitudes

The statement was made above that when consultants (or other program directors) described the objective of a program as ''an attitude change,'' attitudes were considered a stepping stone to a behavioral change; hence one might as well evaluate the behavior itself and omit study of the intervening attitude. A second reason for preferring to evaluate behavior is that in most cases we do not have any empirical basis for assuming that change in a given attitude leads to change in a related behavior, that is, for assuming that the attitude is truly a stepping stone to the behavior. For example, although common sense might lead us to assume that supervisors in a training program who came to have a more ''liberal'' attitude toward the women working for them, as measured by some attitude scale, would also act more ''liberally'' toward the women themselves, we have no proof that such a relationship exists between attitude and behavior. It is my belief, for these reasons, that an evaluator should always assess behavior in any evaluation and that if attitude is to be assessed it should be assessed in conjunction with behavior and not as the sole approach. The evaluation of attitudes has its place but only if accompanied by the evaluation of behavior.

There are three strategies a consultant can use to evaluate attitudes—a generalized scale appropriate for the attitude of almost any concept, the consultant's own attitude scale, or a previously used scale, found in one of the many resource books on attitude scales, assessing the specific attitude of concern. There are two generalized attitude scales: the Semantic Differential and the Adjective Check List. The Semantic Differential consists of a set of bipolar adjectives (e.g., good−bad, strong−weak, hot−cold, and so on); each one of a pair is placed at the opposite end of a seven-point scale. The participant locates the specified concept (e.g., Republicans, job supervisors, and teenage mother) on the scale, placing, for example, Republican exactly midway between good and bad, five points away from hot, and three points away from strong.

A large set of bipolar adjectives was studied by Osgood and Suci (1969) and factor-analyzed into three types of attitudes: evaluation (good−bad, pleasant−unpleasant, fair−unfair), potency (large−small, heavy−light, thick−thin), and activity (sharp−dull, active−passive, fast−slow). The evaluator selects several adjectives from each of the three types to make up the scale so that results can be divided into an evaluation attitude, a potency attitude, and an activity attitude toward the given concept. The Semantic Differential has been used by Zacker, Rutter and Bard (1971) to assess changes in attitudes toward each other of consultants and police officers as a result of a 14-week consultation program. Further examples of its use and the complete set of bipolar adjectives are given by Snider and Osgood (1975).

The Adjective Check List (Gough & Heilbrun, 1965) consists of a series of adjectives appropriate for the description of groups of people (e.g., calm, greedy, meek, responsible, tough). Participants check off all that they think apply. The adjectives have been factor-analyzed by Gough and Heilbrun into various categories (e.g., dominance, order, nurturance, introception, autonomy, counseling readiness, and so on), allowing the evaluator to describe the participants' attitude toward the given groups of people, saying, for example, that the participants perceived the group of psychiatrists as high on dominance before a consultation program on psychiatry and as low on dominance afterwards. Zacker et al. (1971) used the Adjective Check List and found that the consultants perceived the police as less aggressive and more introceptive after the program than before.

The second strategy a consultant can use to evaluate attitudes is to create a new attitude scale: this procedure is not recommended. Consultants who use freshly created scales cannot be certain that they are measuring what the consultants think they are measuring, although the items may appear reasonably related. The process of creating your own scale and proving its validity (or showing that it is really measuring the attitude you want it to measure) is technically complex and logistically time-consuming [for an explanation of the process involved, see Thorndike and Hagen (1969)].

A better solution is to spend some time looking for a scale previously used and validated by someone else. An excellent resource is the series of handbooks of instruments of attitude measurement by Robinson and co-workers (1973; 1973; 1975). The reference book by Shaw and Wright (1967), also contains scales measuring a great diversity of attitudes. All of these reference books describe the work performed previously with each scale and offer critical comments on each scale's validity and reliability.

Consultee Satisfaction

The evaluation approaches discussed up to this point (simulated situations, supervisor and peer ratings, existing agency records, and attitudes) have had as a requirement for their use two implementations, one before and one after the consultation program, in order to assess the impact of the program. While evidence obtained through a ''before–after'' research design is necessary if the consultant is to have any degree of assurance that change was due to the consultation program and not to other factors, the consultant can obtain useful information by having the consultee complete a ''consultee satisfaction'' questionnaire solely at the end of the program. The consultees can tell the consultant what they felt they learned, what additional material they would like to have learned, how useful they found specific consultation training techniques, and so on. A consultee satisfaction form is not a substitute for a before–after evaluation of behavior or attitude; it provides additional useful feedback on the consultees' opinions of various aspects of the program. However, the consultant who cannot do any sort of before–after evaluation should institute a consultee satisfaction questionnaire to obtain some feedback on the program.

The questions on a consultee satisfaction questionnaire are crucial. If the consultant asks the participants to describe "your reaction to the program" they will give such answers as "It was very helpful," "I got a lot out of it," "Most of it was irrelevant to my work," and so on. The questionnaire must contain questions about specific aspects of the program and must be written so that the consultee knows exactly what the consultant wants information about. Tobiessen and Shai (1971), for example, asked teachers who had participated in mental health consultation to answer, "To what extent did the consultation generate discussions and exchange of ideas among teachers in your school?" by checking off on a five-point scale running from "not at all" to "large extent" (p. 220). Scheidlinger, Struening, and Rabkin (1970) asked directors of community agencies that had received consultation to answer a series of specific questions including an opinion of each component of the consultation and a ranking of the components "in order of their importance to the community organizations" (p. 493).

In making up a client satisfaction questionnaire, the consultant should first list all meaningful components of the program, including topics covered, training approaches used (role playing, films, and so on), and scheduling (frequency, regularity, timing), and should then list, in specific terms, all objectives of the program, such as "to generate discussions," "to increase awareness of mothers' emotional states." "to heighten sensitivity to workers' personal problems," and so on. These two lists constitute the areas the consultant wants feedback on, and a question asking about each item on the list should be created.

It is advisable, when reasonable, to ask participants to answer in part by rating the particular item on a scale such as that used by Tobiessen and Shai (1971) which allows the consultant to quickly obtain an overall accurate impression of the responses [see Mariner, Brandt, Stone, and Mirmow (1961) for a description of the results of a client satisfaction questionnaire using rating scales] and to easily compare the responses of two or more separate groups of participants. Participants should also be encouraged to answer each question in a narrative fashion by explaining their ratings; each question might be followed by a subquestion such as "please explain why you rated X as you did."

Occasionally it is difficult to predict all of the possible results of the program and hence to ask about each in a specific question. In this case, the consultant can ask open-ended questions, such as Neff et al. (1975) did in their evaluation of consultation to police managers: they asked, for example, "At this point in time, what (if anything) do you think is the most important thing(s) you're learning from the management training program?" Norman and Forti (1972) describe the results of questions asking the consultees in what ways the consultation had and had not been helpful to them. The answers given to such questions should be categorized in the same manner as the answers in the Critical Incident Technique or in the simulated situation method described above.

An excellent, although rather gross, indicator of client satisfaction is the consultee's request for further consultation. This indicator is recommended by both Barry (1970), in his discussion of the various criteria one can apply in the evaluation of consultation, and Caplan (1970), who feels that such a request is particularly significant when it involves a ''budgetary decision'' (p. 297). Although ideally the evaluation should also incorporate other techniques, one would hope that, on this criterion at least, most consultations succeed.

REFERENCES

Bachrach, L. Uses and limitations of existing data sources in the assessment of unmet health needs: Patient records and service statistics. Paper presented at the XIV Meeting of the National Conference on Mental Health Statistics, sponsored by the National Institute of Mental Health, Washington, D.C., June 1972.

Barry, J. R. Criteria in the evaluation of consultation. *Professional Psychology,* 1970, VI, 363–366.

Behavior Science Corporation. *Evaluation of the impact of community mental health center consultation services on school systems. Volume II: The dynamics of school consultation* (prepared for National Institute of Mental Health.) (NTIS No. PB-225 774, October 1973.)

Berlin, I. N. An effort to update mental health consultation methods. In *Mental health consultation to the schools: Directions for the future* (prepared for National Institute of Mental Health by Behavior Science Corporation) (NTIS No. PB-225 775, May 1973).

Brown, J. W. Pragmatic notes on community consultation with agencies. *Community Mental Health Journal,* 1967, *3,* 339–405.

Caplan, G. *The theory and practice of mental health consultation.* New York: Basic Books, 1970.

Cutler, R. L., & McNeil, E. B. *Mental health consultation in schools: A research analysis.* Ann Arbor: Department of Psychology, University of Michigan, 1966.

Delworth, N., Rudow, E. H., & Taub, J. (Eds.). *Crisis center/hotline: A guidebook to beginning and operating.* Springfield, Ill.: Charles C. Thomas, 1972.

Dorsey, J. R., Matsunaga, G., & Bauman, G. Training public health nurses in mental health. *Archives of General Psychiatry,* 1964, *11,* 214–222.

Flaherty, E. W., & Martin, E. G. The utility of a daily log used at periodic intervals for administration and evaluation. Hahnemann Community Mental Health/Mental Retardation Center, Research and Evaluation Service Report No. 42, 1976.

Flanagan, J. C. The critical incident technique. *Psychological Bulletin,* 1954, *51,* 327–358.

France, K. Evaluation of lay volunteer crisis telephone workers. *American Journal of Community Psychology*, 1975, *3*, 197−220.

Gough, H. G., & Heilbrun, A. B. *The Adjective Check List manual*. Palo Alto: Consulting Psychologists Press, 1965.

Guttentag, M., Kiresuk, T., Oglesby, M., & Cahn, J. *The evaluation of training in mental health*. New York: Behavioral Publications, 1975.

Hargreaves, W. A., Attkisson, C. C., Siegel, L. M., McIntyre, M. H., & Sorensen, J. E. *Resource materials for community mental health program evaluation: Part II−Needs assessment and planning*. Bethesda: National Institute of Mental Health, 1974.

Kahn, R. L., & Cannell, C. F. *The dynamics of interviewing; Theory, technique and cases*. New York: John Wiley & Sons, 1957.

Keutzer, C. S., Fosmire, F. R., Diller, R., & Smith, M. D. Laboratory training in a new social system: Evaluation of a consulting relationship with a high school faculty. *Journal of Applied Behavioral Science*, 1971, *7*, 493−501.

Krebs, R. Using attendance as a means of evaluating community mental health programs. *Community Mental Health Journal*, 1971, *7*, 72−77.

Lane, D. S., & Kelman, H. R. Assessment of material health care quality: Conceptual and methodologic issues. *Medical Care*, 1975, *13*, 791−807.

Mannino, F. V. Perceptions of consultation by consultants and consultees. Bethesda: Mental Health Study Center, National Institute of Mental Health, 1969.

Mannino, F. V. Task accomplishment and consultation outcome. *Community Mental Health Journal*, 1972, *8*, 102−108.

Mariner, A. S., Brandt, E., Stone, E. & Mirmow, E. L. Group psychiatric consultation with public school personnel—a two-year study. *Personnel and Guidance Journal*, 1961, *40*, 254−258.

Miller, N. *Guidelines for evaluation of continuing education programs in mental health*. Washington, D. C.: National Institute of Mental Health, DHEW Publication No. (ADM) 75−224, 1975.

Montague, E. K., & Taylor, E. N. *Handbook on procedures for evaluating mental health indirect service programs in schools*. (Prepared for National Institute of Mental Health, Human Resources Research Organization, August, 1971).

Morgan, J. P., & King, G. D. The selection and evaluation of the volunteer paraprofessional telephone counselor. *American Journal of Community Psychology*, 1975, *3*, 237−249.

Neff, F. W., Lubin, B., & McConnell, K. Impact of training on self-description and co-worker description of police managerial behavior. *American Journal of Community Psychology*, 1975, *3*, 391−402.

Norman, E. C., & Forti, T. J. A study of the process and the outcome of mental health consultation. *Community Mental Health Journal*, 1972, *8*, 261−270.

Osgood, C. E., & Suci, G. J. Factor analysis of meaning. In J. G. Snider & C. E. Osgood (Eds.), *Semantic differential technique: A sourcebook*. Chicago: Aldine Publishing, 1969. Also available in *Journal of Experimental Psychology*, 1955, *50*, 325−338.

Robbins, P. R., Spencer, E. C., & Frank, D. A. Some factors influencing the outcome of consultation. *American Journal of Public Health*, 1970, *60*, 524−534.

Robinson, J. P., Athanasiou, R., & Head, K. B. *Measures of occupational attitudes and occupational characteristics.* Ann Arbor: University of Michigan Institute for Social Research, 1973.

Robinson, J. P., Rusk, J. G., & Head, K. B. *Measures of political attitudes.* Ann Arbor: University of Michigan Institute for Social Research, 1973.

Robinson, J. P., & Shaver, P. R. *Measures of social psychological attitudes.* Ann Arbor: University of Michigan Institute for Social Research, 1975.

St. Clair, C. H., Silver, M. J., & Spivack, G. An instrument to assess staff time utilization in a community mental health center. *Community Mental Health Journal,* 1975, *11,* 371−380.

Scheidlinger, S., Struening, E. L., & Rabkin, J. G. Evaluation of a mental health consultation service in a ghetto area. *American Journal of Psychotherapy,* 1970, *24,* 485−493.

Shaw, M. E., & Wright, J. M. *Scales for the measurement of attitudes.* New York: McGraw-Hill, 1967.

Snider, J. G., & Osgood, C. N. *Semantic differential techniques: A source book.* Chicago, Illinois: Aldine, 1969.

Spivack, G., & Jamison, M. Incidents that affect staff morale in a community mental health/mental retardation center. Hahnemann Community Mental Health/Mental Retardation Center, Research and Evaluation Service Report No. 32, 1975.

Stephenson, P. S. Judging the effectiveness of a consultation program to a community agency. *Community Mental Health Journal,* 1973, *9,* 253−259.

Teese, C. F., & Van Wormer, J. Mental health training and consultation with suburban police. *Community Mental Health Journal.* 1975, *11,* 115−121.

Thorndike, R. L., & Hagen, E. *Measurement and evaluation in psychology and education.* New York: John Wiley & Sons, 1969.

Tobiessen, J., & Shai, A. A comparison of individual and group mental health consultation with teachers. *Community Mental Health Journal,* 1971, *7,* 218−226.

Warheit, G. J., Bell, R. A., & Schwab, J.J. *Planning for change: Needs assessment approaches.* Bethesda: National Institute of Mental Health, 1974.

Webb, E. J., Campbell, D. T., Schwartz, R. D., & Sechrest, L. *Unobtrusive measures.* Chicago, Illinois: Rand McNally College Publishing, 1966.

Wingert, W. A., Grubbs, J., Lenoski, E. F., & Friedman, D. B. Effectiveness and efficiency of indigenous health aides in a pediatric outpatient department. *American Journal of Public Health,* 1975, *65,* 849−857.

Zacker, J., Rutter, E., & Bard, M. Evaluation of attitudinal changes in a program of community consultation. *Community Mental Health Journal,* 1971, *7,* 236−241.

Index

a
b
c
d
e
f
9 g
0 h
1 i
8 2 j